THE VACCINE HANDBOOK

THE VACCINE HANDBOOK

A Practitioner's Guide to Maximizing Use and Efficacy across the Lifespan

Tina Q. Tan, MD
PROFESSOR OF PEDIATRICS
FEINBERG SCHOOL OF MEDICINE
NORTHWESTERN UNIVERSITY
INFECTIOUS DISEASES ATTENDING
ANN AND ROBERT H. LURIE CHILDREN'S HOSPITAL
PRENTICE WOMEN'S HOSPITAL

John P. Flaherty, MD
PROFESSOR OF MEDICINE
FEINBERG SCHOOL OF MEDICINE
NORTHWESTERN UNIVERSITY
INFECTIOUS DISEASES ATTENDING
NORTHWESTERN MEMORIAL HOSPITAL

Melvin V. Gerbie, MD
PROFESSOR EMERITUS OF OBSTETRICS AND GYNECOLOGY
FEINBERG SCHOOL OF MEDICINE
NORTHWESTERN UNIVERSITY
PRENTICE WOMEN'S HOSPITAL

OXFORD
UNIVERSITY PRESS

OXFORD
UNIVERSITY PRESS

Oxford University Press is a department of the University of Oxford. It furthers
the University's objective of excellence in research, scholarship, and education
by publishing worldwide. Oxford is a registered trade mark of Oxford University
Press in the UK and certain other countries.

Published in the United States of America by Oxford University Press
198 Madison Avenue, New York, NY 10016, United States of America.

Library of Congress Cataloging-in-Publication Data
Names: Tan, Tina Q., author. | Flaherty, John P., author. | Gerbie, Melvin V., author.
Title: The vaccine handbook: a practitioner's guide to maximizing use and efficacy across
the lifespan / Tina Q. Tan, John P. Flaherty, Melvin V. Gerbie.
Description: New York, NY : Oxford University Press, [2018] |
Includes bibliographical references.
Identifiers: LCCN 2016036635 (print) | LCCN 2016037351 (ebook) |
ISBN 9780190604776 (pbk. : alk. paper) | ISBN 9780190604783 (UPDF) |
ISBN 9780190604790 (EPUB)
Subjects: | MESH: Vaccination | Immunization Schedule | Handbooks
Classification: LCC RA638 (print) | LCC RA638 (ebook) | NLM QW 39 |
DDC 614.4/7—dc23
LC record available at https://lccn.loc.gov/2016036635

1 3 5 7 9 8 6 4 2
Printed by WebCom, Inc., Canada

CONTENTS

INTRODUCTION

DID YOU KNOW THAT:

- The concept of vaccination and attempts to vaccinate have been traced back to the 7th century when some Indian Buddhists drank snake venom in an attempt to become immune to its effects.
- Immunization is one of the most successful public health initiatives of all time. Each year, immunization prevents an estimated 2 to 3 million deaths from diphtheria, tetanus, pertussis, and measles worldwide. These are all life-threatening diseases that disproportionately affect children.
- Immunization was critical in the eradication of smallpox and the near eradication of polio.
- One out of 5 infants worldwide (20% of children) remains unprotected against common vaccine preventable

diseases—over 70% live in 10 countries: Afghanistan, Chad, the Democratic Republic of Congo, Ethiopia, India, Indonesia, Nigeria, Pakistan, the Philippines, and South Africa.

The development of vaccines against multiple infectious diseases is one of the greatest public health achievements of the past century. Infant and childhood vaccination rates are high in the United States; however, vaccination rates in the adolescent and the adult populations are still below the Healthy People 2020 goals, leaving much room for improvement. Vaccine preventable diseases (VPDs) still cause 50,000 to 90,000 deaths and hundreds of thousands of hospitalizations in adults each year in the United States. This poses a major public health problem to everyone in the community, especially to young infants that are either too young to be immunized or who are incompletely immunized. To protect against these VPDs, an increasing number of preventative vaccines are recommended for routine administration to persons of all ages.

So what makes this book different? This book covers the majority of vaccine issues and provides answers to common questions that a busy healthcare provider may encounter on a daily basis presented in a practical, easy-to-understand format. The book can easily be carried in a lab-coat pocket or can be quickly accessed from office or clinic shelves to provide ready answers to common issues. This book is written so that healthcare providers in different specialties and at all levels of training and practice can optimally recommend the appropriate vaccines for their patients of any age. There are several comprehensive textbooks covering all aspects of vaccinology in great detail, but these books are not formatted as a quick, readily accessible reference while seeing patients in an office, clinic, or on patient rounds.

Today, the practice of medicine requires healthcare providers to obtain and record more comprehensive patient information, including complete vaccination histories on their patients. This book is written to assist all providers in not only obtaining vaccine histories but also to provide guidance in recommending and administering the currently recommended vaccines for age according to CDC guidelines. The book also has a section on addressing and speaking with vaccine-hesitant patients, which is encountered more frequently by healthcare providers in all areas of medicine. Storage and procedural issues are well covered in this book and provide guidance for healthcare providers taking care of patients of any age.

As our world shrinks, and as international travel becomes easier, more widespread, and affordable, many vaccine-preventable diseases that are still endemic in other countries are now just a plane, boat, car, or bus ride away. Individuals who travel to these countries and are not appropriately vaccinated can contract these diseases and become ill while traveling or bring the disease back home, serving as a nidus for spread to other citizens. This handbook provides guidance to the healthcare provider in preparing patients who are planning to travel to countries abroad to protect them against various diseases.

Also the "Did You Know That" sections at the beginning of each chapter provide interesting information about the vaccines and vaccine-preventable diseases.

A major barrier to vaccine usage, especially in the adult population, is a widespread lack of understanding among healthcare providers caring primarily for adults concerning

- the importance of preventative vaccines in their patients
- the diseases against which the preventative vaccines provide protection

- the population for whom the vaccines are indicated
- cost issues and reimbursement
- responsibility for providing vaccine information and vaccine access to their patients

Solutions to these barriers are addressed in the book.

We invite you to explore this practical and easy-to-understand handbook and hope that you will find the information useful in (1) gaining a better understanding of why preventative vaccination should be an integral part of routine healthcare at all ages, (2) providing some suggestions to help you to talk to your patients about vaccines, and (3) arming you with the information needed so that you can provide the recommended vaccinations to them.

We look forward to any thoughts and suggestions that you may have in helping us to improve this handbook.

Tina Q. Tan, M.D.
John P. Flaherty, M.D.
Melvin V. Gerbie, M.D.

PART I

VACCINE OVERVIEW

VACCINE FACTS

- **Active immunization** involves the administration of all or part of a microorganism or a modified product of a microorganism (a toxoid, a purified antigen, or an antigen produced by genetic engineering) to evoke an immunologic response that mimics that of natural infection.
- **Passive immunization** involves the administration of preformed antibody to a recipient and achieves protection only for a short period of time (IM immunoglobulin or intravenous immunoglobulin—IVIG).
- Vaccines may be **inactivated** or **live, attenuated**. Inactivated vaccines are composed of inactivated whole cells or particles that are unable to multiply. These vaccines function by stimulating humoral immune responses and by priming for immunological memory. With live attenuated vaccines, there is active replication of the organism in the host that produces a modified infection to which the host develops an immune response.
- The **immunologic response to a vaccine** is dependent on the type and dose of antigen, the effect of adjuvants (materials added to a vaccine to improve the immune response

1

to the antigen [aluminum salts]), and host factors related to age, preexisting antibody, nutrition, concurrent disease, immune status, or drug effect and genetics of the host.

- Some vaccines provide nearly complete and lifelong protection against disease, others provide partial protection, and some need to be given at regular intervals to maintain disease protection.
- Two or more inactivated vaccines may be administered simultaneously in different sites.
- Inactivated and live vaccines may be administered simultaneously (Tdap and intranasal influenza).
- Two or more live vaccines may be administered simultaneously at the **same** visit.
- A **break** in the **immunization schedule of a vaccine** does *not* **require starting the entire series over** or **giving additional doses** of the vaccine. If a dose of vaccine is missed, subsequent immunization should be given at the next visit as if the usual interval between doses had elapsed.
- **Live, attenuated vaccines** are **contraindicated** in persons who are **pregnant** and those **with known or suspected immunodeficiency** (there are some exceptions).

The Advisory Committee on Immunization Practices (ACIP) of the Centers for Disease Control and Prevention (CDC) now designates a **vaccine recommendation as either "A" or "B."**

- An **"A"** recommendation means the vaccine is routinely recommended for all children and adults in an age or risk group.
- A **"B"** recommendation means that the vaccine is for permissive use at the discretion of the clinician or health-care provider.

The Affordable Care Act requires insurance plans to provide benefit coverage of vaccines with both A and B recommendations. The Vaccines for Children (VFC) program also includes vaccines with a "B" recommendation.

ADDRESSING PATIENT CONCERNS ABOUT RECEIVING VACCINES

Vaccines are one of the greatest public health achievements of modern medicine. In the early 20th century, before the routine use of vaccines, about 1 in 6 children under 5 years of age died of a vaccine-preventable disease, especially diseases such as measles, smallpox, pertussis, or rubella. Vaccination programs have contributed significantly to the marked decline in morbidity and mortality of various vaccine-preventable diseases and are credited with the worldwide eradication of smallpox and the virtual elimination of polio from many areas of the world. However, concerns about the safety of vaccines and hesitancy to receive vaccines have been voiced since the introduction of vaccines to the public. For example, Benjamin Franklin's son, Francis Folger Franklin, died at age 4 of smallpox. The following is a quote from Franklin expressing his profound regret for not immunizing his son and his advice to parents regarding vaccination: "In 1736 I lost one of my sons, a fine boy of four years old, by the small-pox, taken in the common way. I long regretted bitterly, and still regret that I had not given it to him by inoculation. This I mention for the sake of parents who omit that operation, on the supposition that they should never forgive themselves if a child died under it; my example showing that the regret may be the same either way, and that, therefore, the safer should be chosen."

There is a plethora of information on vaccine safety that is available from multiple sources. As patients search the Internet for information on vaccines, they frequently encounter information from poorly designed and conducted studies, misleading information from well-conducted studies, anecdotes, or personal testimonies that are incorrectly written or written to look like real science and that claim vaccines cause autism and are associated with experimentation, are not effective, and in many cases are associated with devastating side effects. Addressing these concerns and fears during a routine health evaluation may be time consuming and stressful for both the health-care provider and the patient (see Table 1). Health-care providers play a key role in establishing and maintaining a commitment to effectively communicating with patients about the importance of vaccines and maintaining high vaccination rates. We must remember that a successful discussion about vaccines involves a two-way conversation, with both parties sharing information and asking questions. Important principles to bring to the discussion include: taking time to listen (this can play a major role in helping patients with their decisions to choose vaccination) and soliciting and welcoming questions and concerns—these simple principles go a long way in connecting with patients and facilitating a productive dialogue (Dube et al., 2015; Witteman, 2015).

Studies have shown that most adults do believe that vaccines are important, and a health-care provider's recommendation is the critical factor in whether patients receive the vaccines that they and/or their children need. Recommendation of a vaccine by a health-care provider prompts most patients to get immunized.

However, for some patients, a strong, clear vaccine recommendation may not be enough. The health-care provider can encourage these patients to make an informed decision about vaccination by sharing critical information with them. Based on the

Table 1 BARRIERS TO ADOLESCENT AND ADULT IMMUNIZATION

Patient barriers	Physician barriers
• lack of awareness of disease and associated morbidity	• lack of organized vaccine administration infrastructure
• perception that vaccine has no value and is ineffective	• lack of understanding of importance of vaccines
• perception of low risk for disease	• lack of understanding of the diseases the vaccines protect against and the population for whom vaccines are recommended
• perception that vaccines are experimental and may be dangerous	
• lack of access to vaccines	• lack of awareness of vaccine recommendations
• immunization costs	• discomfort using vaccines
• requirement for multiple doses	• missed opportunities and patient refusal
• perceived vaccine risks and fears of side effects (e.g., developing autism)	• time limitations and patient refusal
• lack of vaccination records	• perception that it is another primary health-care provider's responsibility
• time limitations	• vaccine costs and reimbursement
• perception that getting natural disease is better than receiving vaccine	• inability to verify previous vaccination records
	• storage requirements

CDC SHARE program, the steps to discussing vaccines with these patients includes:

1. **Sharing** the reasons why the recommended vaccine is appropriate for the patient based on their age, health status, lifestyle, occupation, or other factors that place them at risk for a disease.
2. **Highlighting** positive experiences with vaccines to reinforce the benefits and strengthen confidence in vaccination.
3. **Addressing** all patient questions and concerns about the vaccine, including potential side effects, safety, and vaccine effectiveness in easy-to-understand language.
4. **Reminding** patients that vaccines protect them and their families from many common and serious diseases.
5. **Explaining** the potential costs associated with getting the disease, including serious complications, time lost from missing work or family obligations, and the financial costs.

The following are common misconceptions regarding vaccines that patients may express and strategies for addressing these issues.

Misconception #1: Vaccines cause autism

The widespread fear that vaccines increased the risk for autism originated with a 1997 study published in *The Lancet* by Andrew Wakefield, a British gastroenterologist. His study in a small number of children suggested that measles, mumps, rubella (MMR) vaccine was the cause of the increasing amount of autism that was being seen in British children. Further scientific review of the data led to the paper being completely discredited, and the

paper was retracted due to serious procedural errors, ethical viola-
tions, false reporting of data, and undisclosed financial conflicts
of interest. Ultimately, Andrew Wakefield lost his medical license.
However, his hypothesis (which is completely false) continues to
be taken seriously by some people in the community. Multiple
major studies have been conducted, and none have found a link
between any vaccine and the likelihood of developing autism.

The issue of whether vaccines cause autism spectrum disorder (ASD) has been studied extensively, including several
very thorough reviews by the Institute of Medicine (IOM,
2004). A 2004 scientific review by the IOM concluded that
"the evidence favors rejection of a causal relationship between
thimerosal–containing vaccines and ASD" (IOM, 2011). Since
2003 there have been nine CDC-funded or -conducted studies
that have found no link between thimerosal-containing vaccines and ASD and no link between the measles, mumps, and
rubella (MMR) vaccine and ASD in children (DeStefano et al.,
2013). In 2011 an IOM report on eight routinely used vaccines
(MMR, Hepatitis A, meningococcal, varicella zoster, influenza,
Hepatitis B, HPV and tetanus containing vaccines) given to children and adults found that these vaccines are very safe and that
there is no link between receiving vaccines and developing ASD.
A 2013 CDC study added to the research showing that vaccines
do not cause ASD. The study looked at the number of antigens
(substances in vaccines that cause the body's immune system to
produce disease-fighting antibodies) from vaccines during the
first two years of life. The results showed that the total amount
of antigen from vaccines received was the same between children with ASD and those that did not have ASD. All the extensive research performed to date shows absolutely no evidence of
any link between receiving vaccines or those vaccines containing
trace thimerosal and ASD.

The true causes of autism are probably multifactorial but have no link to vaccines. Several recent studies have now identified symptoms of autism in children well before they receive the MMR vaccine, and others provide evidence that autism may develop in utero well before the baby is born or receives any vaccines.

Health-care provider communication tips

When patients raise concerns and hypotheses linking vaccines to autism, there are 4 items critical in addressing these issues:

a. The health-care provider should provide the patient with empathetic reassurance that he/she understands that the patient's health or their child's health is the patient's top priority and that it is also the health-care provider's top priority to ensure that putting the patient or their child at risk of vaccine-preventable diseases without any scientific evidence of a link between vaccines and autism is a risk that the health-care provider is not willing to take

b. Acknowledge that the onset of symptoms of autism spectrum disorder is known to often coincide with the timing of vaccines but is in no way caused by vaccines. Offer to share information from well-designed and well-conducted studies that show that MMR and other vaccines do not cause autism.

c. Emphasize that as a health-care provider, your personal and professional opinion is that vaccines are very safe and are important in protecting against potentially serious infections.

d. Remind the patient that vaccine preventable diseases may cause serious complications and even death and that these diseases are still present and remain a threat.

Misconception #2: An infant's immune system becomes overwhelmed and cannot handle the number of vaccines given

Infant immune systems are much stronger than one might imagine. Neonates develop the capacity to respond to foreign antigens before they are born. B and T cells are present by 14 weeks' gestation and express an enormous array of antigen-specific receptors. Based on the number of antibodies present in the blood, an infant would theoretically have the ability to respond to around 10,000 vaccines at one time. So even if all the doses of the scheduled vaccines during the first 5 years of life were given at once, it would only "use up" about 0.1% (1/10th of 1%) of an infant's immune capacity. The immune system can never really be overwhelmed given that the cells in the system are constantly being replenished (e.g., 2 billion CD4+ T lymphocytes are replenished on a daily basis). In reality, infants are exposed to countless numbers (tens of thousands) of bacteria and viruses on a daily basis through the activities of daily living in their environment (e.g., daycare, going to the park, the grocery store, the mall, playdates etc), and the number of antigens in routine immunizations are negligible in comparison (Offit, Quarles, et al., 2002).

Health-care provider communication tips
Parents/patients may bring up concerns of receiving more than one vaccine at a time, having a strong preference of receiving vaccines at a later time, and/or receiving vaccines on an alternative schedule with regard to timing and spacing of vaccines that is different from the recommended schedule. It is important to emphasize that:

a. The routine vaccine schedules are designed to provide protection at the earliest possible time against serious diseases that may affect a person early in life. The timing of when the vaccines are administered in the routine schedule has been extensively studied and provides the optimal immune protection against a disease. Using alternative schedules is very strongly discouraged since it is unknown if a person will develop protective immunity against a disease by receiving vaccines by these schedules.

b. Vaccine-preventable diseases may be associated with serious morbidity and mortality that is prevented by vaccines.

c. Each vaccine series should be started on time to protect patients (especially infants and children) as soon as possible, and each multidose series must be completed to provide the best protection against a disease. Receiving only 1 dose of a multidose series does not provide adequate protective immunity.

Misconception #3: Natural immunity is better than vaccine-acquired immunity and vaccines are more dangerous than the diseases they prevent

Most people may not have seen or heard firsthand of a case of a vaccine-preventable disease because of the effectiveness of the vaccines that are used today. Therefore, many people assume that the disease is no longer present and question whether vaccines are really needed. They may also believe that the risks of being vaccinated far outweigh the benefits of protecting them from infection caused by vaccine-preventable diseases.

In a small number of cases, natural immunity—defined as actually contracting the disease and becoming ill—may result in a stronger immune response to the disease than a vaccination. However, the dangers of this approach far outweigh any possible relative benefits. For example, if you wanted to develop immunity to measles by contracting the disease, you have a 1 in 500 chance of dying from your disease. In contrast, the number of people who have had severe allergic reactions from an MMR vaccine is less than 1 in 1 million. Likewise, a natural chickenpox infection may result in pneumonia, bacterial skin infections, or necrotizing fasciitis, whereas, the varicella vaccine may only cause a sore arm or leg for a couple of days.

Health-care provider communication tips
   a. Provide information from your own experience about the seriousness of the vaccine preventable diseases (e.g., complications from influenza, pneumococcal disease, varicella, herpes zoster).
   b. Explain that there continue to be cases and outbreaks of vaccine-preventable diseases occurring now in the United States, and that even when diseases have been eliminated in the United States they can make a rapid return in unimmunized infants, children, and adults who are exposed to another unimmunized person with the disease, or if they travel abroad, contract the disease, and bring it back to the United States.
   c. Any vaccine-preventable disease can strike at any time in the United States because all of these diseases still circulate either in the United States or elsewhere in the world. A vaccine-preventable disease is only a plane, train, bus, boat, or car ride away.

Misconception #4: Vaccines contain harmful toxins

Fears over the safety of vaccines have substantially increased over the last 3 decades. Concerns have grown over the use of formaldehyde, mercury, or aluminum in vaccines. It is true that high levels of these chemicals are toxic to the human body; however, only minute trace amounts of some of these chemicals are used in FDA-approved vaccines. For example, the amount of formaldehyde produced by our own metabolic systems is much higher than that used in vaccines, and there is no evidence that low levels of this chemical, mercury, or aluminum in vaccines are harmful.

Questions regarding whether a vaccine contains thimerosal continue to arise. Thimerosal is an ethylmercury containing organic compound (organomercurial) that, since the 1930s, has been used widely as a preservative in a number of biological and drug products, including multidose vials of vaccines, to help prevent potentially life threatening contamination with harmful microbes. Because of an increasing awareness of the theoretical potential for neurotoxicity of low levels of organomercurials, and the increased number of thimerosal containing vaccines that had been added to the infant immunization schedule, concerns about the use of thimerosal in vaccines and other products have been raised. The Food and Drug Administration (FDA) continues to work with vaccine manufacturers to reduce or completely eliminate thimerosal from vaccines.

Thimerosal has been removed from or reduced to trace amounts (remaining as a part of the manufacturing process and defined as 1 microgram or less of organomercury per dose) in all vaccines routinely recommended for children 6 years of age and younger, with the exception of a specific influenza vaccine. Preservative free versions of the inactivated influenza vaccine and Td vaccine (both which contain trace amounts of thimerosal) are available.

Table 2 shows those vaccines in multidose vials that contain some thimerosal.

Table 2 VACCINES CONTAINING THIMEROSAL

Vaccine	Brand	Manufacturer	Thimerosal concentration	Mercury mcg/0.5 mL
Tetanus toxoid	Generic	Sanofi Pasteur	0.01%	25
Influenza inactivated	Afluria	CSL limited for Merck	0.01%	24.5
	FluLaval Quadrivalent	GlaxoSmithKline	0.01%	25
	Fluvirin	Novartis	0.01%	25
	Fluzone	Sanofi Pasteur	0.01%	25

Health-care provider communication tips

a. Remind patients that there are ongoing efforts by the CDC and FDA to ensure the safety of the vaccines that are currently used and that the vaccines used today are the safest that they have ever been.

b. Explain that multiple years of study of the various ingredients contained in vaccines (e.g., thimerosal, aluminum, gelatin, human serum albumin, formaldehyde, antibiotics, egg proteins, and yeast proteins) have not been found to be harmful in humans or experimental animals. The content of these agents are minute and are used to prevent bacterial or fungal contamination (e.g., thimerosal); enhance antigen-specific immune responses (e.g., aluminum salts); stabilize live, attenuated viral vaccines (e.g., gelatin, human serum albumin) or are residuals from the manufacturing process (e.g., formaldehyde, antibiotics, egg proteins, and yeast proteins) (Offit, Jew, 2003).

REFERENCES

1) Institute for vaccine safety. www.vaccinesafety.edu
2) CDC. Thimerosal in vaccines. http://www.cdc.gov/vaccinesafety/concerns/thimerosal/
3) U.S. Food and Drug Administration. Thimerosal in vaccines. http://www.fda.gov/BiologicsBloodVaccines/SafetyAvailability/VaccineSafety/UCM0962

Misconception #5: The development of better hygiene and sanitation, nutrition, and the development of antibiotics are actually responsible for decreasing the number of vaccine preventable infections—not the vaccines themselves

These developments all contributed to reducing rates of infectious diseases; however, when these factors are taken in isolation, their impact on the rates of vaccine-preventable infectious diseases is low compared to when vaccines are factored into the equation. The routine use of vaccines has had a substantial impact on the incidence of vaccine preventable diseases and has resulted in the eradication of smallpox worldwide. An example of the impact of vaccine is *Haemophilus influenzae* type b disease (Hib). Prior to the introduction of effective Hib conjugate vaccines in the early 1990s, Hib was the most common case of bacterial meningitis and invasive bacterial disease in the United States in children under 5 years of age. In 1990 there were 20,000 cases of invasive Hib disease. This number markedly declined to about 1,500 cases in 1993, following the introduction of the vaccine. With routine use of conjugate Hib vaccines, the incidence of Hib disease has decreased by 99% to fewer than 1 case per 100,000 children younger than 5 years of age. There were no significant changes in hygiene, sanitation, and nutrition during this time period. Today in the United States, invasive Hib disease occurs primarily in unimmunized or underimmunized children and among infants too young to have completed the primary immunization series. Hib remains an important pathogen in many resource-limited countries where Hib vaccines are not routinely available.

Health-care provider communication tips

    a. Provide some of the above information to your patients so that they have an understanding of the role that vaccines play in reducing and eliminating the incidence of vaccine preventable diseases.

Misconception #6: Vaccines are not worth the risk

Despite parental concerns, children have been successfully vaccinated for decades. There has never been a single credible study linking vaccines to long-term health conditions. It is also important for the patient to realize that by not being vaccinated, they place themselves and/or their children at risk for contracting a vaccine-preventable disease that may have serious consequences. Patients need to be aware that the presentation of these diseases can range from mild to severe and life-threatening, and there is no way to know beforehand if a person will get a mild or serious case.

As long as a large majority (85% to 99%) of people are immunized in any population (herd immunity), even the unimmunized minority will be protected against a disease. This prevents a disease from being transmitted and spreading within the population. This is important because there will always be a portion of the population—young infants, pregnant women, elderly, and those with immunocompromising conditions—that cannot receive vaccines. However, if too many people fail to vaccinate themselves or their children, they contribute to an increasing danger that opens up opportunities for viruses and bacteria to reestablish themselves in a community and spread. For example, international travel is rapidly growing. Even if a disease is not a threat in the United States, it may be common in other countries that do not routinely vaccinate against the disease. If someone from that country were to carry the disease into the United States from abroad, or if an unvaccinated individual were to travel to that country and contract the disease, other unvaccinated individuals in the United States would be at a far greater risk of getting sick if they were exposed.

Health-care provider communication tips
When patients make the decision to delay or reject vaccines, they need to understand that there are responsibilities that they need to take that could impact their life, their child's life, or the life of someone else. They need to understand the following:

a. If they are ill or their child is ill and they visit the doctor, clinic, or a hospital emergency room, call 911, or ride in an ambulance, they must inform the medical staff that they or their child is unvaccinated or has not received all the recommended age-specific vaccines.

b. Telling health-care personnel their vaccination status or their child's vaccination status is critical for several reasons:

   i. The treating physician will need to consider the possibility that the person has a vaccine-preventable disease as the cause of their illness.

ii. The persons helping that patient or their child can take precautions (e.g., patient can be placed in isolation) so that the disease does not spread to others, especially those patients in high-risk groups that are either too young to be vaccinated or cannot be vaccinated due to an underlying condition.

Misconception #7: Vaccines can cause the disease that they are trying to prevent

Vaccines can cause mild symptoms that may resemble those of the disease they are protecting against. A common misconception is that these symptoms indicate an infection when, in fact, in the small percentage of cases where patients develop symptoms after the vaccine, it is the patient's own immune response to the vaccine and not an infection that is causing the symptoms.

Health-care provider communication tips

If your patients are searching the Internet for basic information on vaccines, recommend they seek websites that are recommended by a credible source, whose information is updated on a regular basis, and whose content is researched, written, and approved by subject matter experts, including physicians, researchers, epidemiologists, and analysts. Reliable sources of vaccine information that you can use and direct your patient to include the following:

a. American Academy of Pediatrics (http://www2.aap.org/immunizations/families/evaluatingwebinfo.html)

b. Immunization Action Coalition (http://www.vaccineinformation.org/internet-immunization-info/)

c. National Network for Immunization Information (NNii)
(http://www.immunizationinfo.org/parents/evaluating-
information-web)
d. Medical Library Association (http://www.mlanet.org

Table 3 COMMON VACCINES BY TYPE

Inactivated Vaccines	Live, Attenuated Vaccines
Td (tetanus and diphtheria)	MMR (measles, mumps, rubella)
Tdap (tetanus, diphtheria, acellular pertussis)	Varicella
Injectable influenza	Intranasal influenza
Hepatitis A	Herpes zoster
Hepatitis B	Rotavirus (infants)
HPV (human papillomavirus)	Oral typhoid fever
IPV (inactivated poliovirus)	Yellow fever
Pneumococcal polysaccharide (PPSV23)	Oral cholera
Pneumococcal conjugate (PCV13)	
Meningococcal conjugate (MCV4)	
Meningococcal B	
Injectable typhoid fever	
Japanese encephalitis	
Rabies	

Table 4 ADMINISTERING VACCINES: DOSE, ROUTE, AND SITE

Vaccine	Dose	Route of Administration
Cholera	3 fluid ounces	Oral
Diphtheria, Tetanus, Pertussis (DTaP, DT, Tdap, Td)	0.5 mL	Intramuscular (IM)
Haemophilus influenzae type b (Hib)	0.5 mL	IM
Hepatitis A (Hep A)	≤ 18 years: 0.5 mL ≥ 19 years: 1.0 mL	IM
Hepatitis B (Hep B)	≤ 19 years: 0.5 mL ≥ 20 years: 1.0 mL	IM
Human papillomavirus (HPV)	0.5 mL	IM
Influenza: live, attenuated (LAIV)	0.2 mL (0.1 mL in each nostril)	Intranasal spray
Influenza: inactivated (IIV); recombinant (RIV) for ages 18 years and older	6 to 35 months: 0.25 mL ≥ 3 years: 0.5 mL	IM
Influenza: inactivated (IIV) Intradermal for ages 18 through 64 years	0.1 mL	Intradermal (ID)
Measles, Mumps, Rubella (MMR)	0.5 mL	Subcutaneous (SC)
Meningococcal conjugate (MCV4 [MenACWY])	0.5 mL	IM

(*continued*)

Table 4 CONTINUED

Vaccine	Dose	Route of Administration
Meningococcal serogroup B (MenB)	0.5 mL	IM
Meningococcal polysaccharide (MPSV)	0.5 mL	SC
Pneumococcal conjugate (PCV)	0.5 mL	IM
Pneumococcal polysaccharide (PPSV23)	0.5 mL	IM or SC
Polio, inactivated (IPV)	0.5 mL	IM or SC
Rotavirus (RV)	Rotarix (RV1): 1.0 mL	Oral
	Rotateq (RV5): 2.0 mL	
Varicella	0.5 mL	SC
Zoster	0.5 mL	SC
Combination vaccines		
DTaP-IPV-Hep B (Pediarix)	0.5 mL	IM
DTaP-IPB-Hib (Pentacel)		
DTaP-IPV (Kinrix; Quadracel)		
Hib-HepB (Comvax)		
Hib-MenCY (MenHibrix)		
MMRV (Proquad)	≤ 12 years: 0.5 mL	SC
HepA-HepB (Twinrix)	≥18 years: 1.0 mL	IM

Table 5 INJECTION SITE AND NEEDLE SIZE

Subcutaneous (SC) Injection—*use a 23- to 25-gauge needle. Choose the injection site that is appropriate for the person's age and body mass.*

Age	Needle Length	Injection site
Infants 1 to 12 months	5/8"	Fatty tissue over anterolateral thigh muscle
Children 12 months and older, adolescents, and adults	5/8"	Fatty tissue over anterolateral thigh muscle or fatty tissues over triceps

Intramuscular (IM) Injection—*use a 22- to 25-gauge needle. Choose the injection site and needle length that is appropriate to the person's age and body mass.*

Age	Needle Length	Injection site
Newborns (1st 28 days)	5/8"	Anterolateral thigh muscle
Infants (1–12 months)	1"	Anterolateral thigh muscle
Toddlers (1–2 years)	1 to 1¼"	Anterolateral thigh muscle or
	5/8" to 1"	Deltoid muscle of arm
Children and teenagers (3–18 years)	5/8" to 1" 1" to 1¼"	Deltoid muscle of arm
Adults 19 years and older		
Female or male < 130 lbs	5/8–1"	Deltoid muscle of arm
Female or male 130–152 lbs	1"	Deltoid muscle of arm
Female 153–200 lbs Male 130–260 lbs	1–1.5"	Deltoid muscle of arm
Female ≥ 200 lbs Male ≥ 260 lbs	1.5"	Deltoid muscle of arm

PART II

VACCINES THROUGHOUT
THE LIFECYCLE

2016 INFANT, CHILD, AND ADOLESCENT IMMUNIZATION SCHEDULES

These recommendations must be read with the footnotes that follow. For those who fall behind or start late, provide catch-up vaccination at the earliest opportunity as indicated by the green bars in Figure 1. To determine minimum intervals between doses, see the catch-up schedule (Figure 2). School entry and adolescent vaccine age groups are shaded.

Vaccine	Birth	1 mo	2 mos	4 mos	6 mos	9 mos	12 mos	15 mos	18 mos	19-23 mos	2-3 yrs	4-6 yrs	7-10 yrs	11-12 yrs	13-15 yrs	16-18 yrs
Hepatitis B[1] (HepB)	1st dose	←2nd dose→			←————— 3rd dose —————→											
Rotavirus[2] (RV) RV1 (2-dose series); RV5 (3-dose series)			1st dose	2nd dose	See footnote 2											
Diphtheria, tetanus, & acellular pertussis[3] (DTaP: <7 yrs)			1st dose	2nd dose	3rd dose		←————— 4th dose —————→					5th dose				
Haemophilus influenzae type b[4] (Hib)			1st dose	2nd dose	See footnote 4		3rd or 4th dose, See footnote 4									
Pneumococcal conjugate[5] (PCV13)			1st dose	2nd dose	3rd dose		←————— 4th dose —————→									
Inactivated poliovirus[6] (IPV: <18 yrs)			1st dose	2nd dose	←————— 3rd dose —————→							4th dose				
Influenza[7] (IIV; LAIV)							Annual vaccination (IIV only) 1 or 2 doses				Annual vaccination (LAIV or IIV) 1 or 2 doses			Annual vaccination (LAIV or IIV) 1 dose only		
Measles, mumps, rubella[8] (MMR)					See footnote 8		←————— 1st dose —————→					2nd dose				
Varicella[9] (VAR)							←————— 1st dose —————→					2nd dose				
Hepatitis A[10] (HepA)							2-dose series, See footnote 10									
Meningococcal[11] (Hib-MenCY ≥6 weeks; MenACWY-D ≥9 mos; MenACWY-CRM ≥2 mos)					See footnote 11									1st dose		(booster)
Tetanus, diphtheria, & acellular pertussis[12] (Tdap: ≥7 yrs)														(Tdap)		
Human papillomavirus[13] (2vHPV: females only; 4vHPV, 9vHPV: males and females)														(3-dose series)		
Meningococcal B[14]														See footnote 11		
Pneumococcal polysaccharide[15] (PPSV23)													See footnote 5			

Legend:
- Range of recommended ages for all children
- Range of recommended ages for catch-up immunization
- Range of recommended ages for certain high-risk groups
- Range of recommended ages for non-high-risk groups that may receive vaccine, subject to individual clinical decision making
- No recommendation

This schedule includes recommendations in effect as of January 1, 2016. Any dose not administered at the recommended age should be administered at a subsequent visit, when indicated and feasible. The use of a combination vaccine generally is preferred over separate injections of its equivalent component vaccines. Vaccination providers should consult the relevant Advisory Committee on Immunization Practices (ACIP) statement for detailed recommendations, available online at http://www.cdc.gov/vaccines/hcp/acip-recs/index.html. Clinically significant adverse events that follow vaccination should be reported to the Vaccine Adverse Event Reporting System (VAERS) online (http://www.vaers.hhs.gov/) or by telephone (800-822-7967). Suspected cases of vaccine-preventable diseases should be reported to the state or local health department. Additional information, including precautions and contraindications for vaccination, is available from CDC online (http://www.cdc.gov/vaccines/recs/vac-admin/contraindications.htm) or by telephone (800-CDC-INFO [800-232-4636]).

This schedule is approved by the Advisory Committee on Immunization Practices (http://www.cdc.gov/vaccines/acip), the American Academy of Pediatrics (http://www.aap.org), the American Academy of Family Physicians (http://www.aafp.org), and the American College of Obstetricians and Gynecologists (http://www.acog.org).

NOTE: The above recommendations must be read along with the footnotes of this schedule (Figure 3).

Figure 1 For those who fall behind or start late, provide catch-up vaccination at the earliest opportunity as indicated in Figure 1

The figure below provides catch-up schedules and minimum intervals between doses for children whose vaccinations have been delayed. A vaccine series does not need to be restarted, regardless of the time that has elapsed between doses. Use the section appropriate for the child's age. Always use this table in conjunction with Figure 1 and the footnotes that follow.

Vaccine	Minimum Age for Dose 1	Children age 4 months through 6 years			
		Minimum Interval Between Doses			
		Does 1 to Dose 2	Dose 2 to Dose 3	Dose 3 to Dose 4	Dose 4 to Dose 5
Hepatitis B[1]	Birth	4 weeks	8 weeks *and* at least 16 weeks after first dose. Minimum age for the final dose is 24 weeks.		
Rotavirus[2]	6 weeks	4 weeks	4 weeks[2]		
Diphtheria, tetanus, and acellular pertussis[3]	6 weeks	4 weeks	4 weeks	6 months	6 months[3]
Haemophilus influenzae type b[4]	6 weeks	4 weeks if first dose was administered before the 1st birthday. 8 weeks (as final dose) if first dose was administered at age 12 through 14 months. No further doses needed if first dose was administered at age 15 months or older.	4 weeks[4] if current age is younger than 12 months **and** first dose was administered at younger than age 7 months, **and** at least 1 previous dose was PRP-T (ActHib, Pentacel) or unknown. 8 weeks *and* age 12 through 59 months (as final dose)[4] • if current age is younger than 12 months **and** first dose was administered at age 7 through 11 months (wait until at least 12 months old); OR	8 weeks (as final dose) This dose only necessary for children age 12 through 59 months who received 3 doses before the 1st birthday.	

Figure 2 Catch up immunization schedule for persons 4 months through 18 years

Vaccine	Minimum age for dose 1	Dose 1 to dose 2	Dose 2 to dose 3	Dose 3 to dose 4
			• if current age is 12 through 59 months **and** first dose was administered before the 1st birthday, **and** second dose administered at younger than 15 months; OR • if both doses were PRP-OMP (PedvaxHIB; Comvax) **and** were administered before the 1st birthday (wait until at least 12 months old). No further doses needed if previous dose was administered at age 15 months or older.	
Pneumococcal[5]	6 weeks	4 weeks if first dose administered before the 1st birthday. 8 weeks (as final dose for healthy children) if first dose was administered at the 1st birthday or after. No further doses needed for healthy children if first dose administered at age 24 months or older.	4 weeks if current age is younger than 12 months and previous dose given at <7months old. 8 weeks (as final dose for healthy children) if previous dose given between 7–11 months (wait until at least 12 months old); OR if current age is 12 months or older and at least 1 dose was given before age 12 months. No further doses needed for healthy children if previous dose administered at age 24 months or older.	8 weeks (as final dose) This dose only necessary for children aged 12 through 59 months who received 3 doses before age 12 months or for children at high risk who received 3 doses at any age.
Inactivated poliovirus[6]	6 weeks	4 weeks[6]	4 weeks[6]	6 months[6] (minimum age 4 years for final dose).
Measles, mumps, rubella[8]	12 months	4 weeks		
Varicella[9]	12 months	3 months		

Vaccine				
Hepatitis A[10]	12 months	6 months	See footnote 11	See footnote 11
Meningococcal[11] (Hib-MenCY ≥ 6 weeks; MenACWY-D ≥ 9 mos); MenACWY-CRM ≥ 2 mos)	6 weeks	8 weeks[11]	See footnote 11	See footnote 11
Children and adolescents age 7 through 18 years				
Meningococcal[11] (Hib-MenCY ≥ 6 weeks; MenACWY-D ≥ 9 mos; MenACWY-CRM ≥ 2 mos)	Not applicable (N/A)	8 weeks[11]		
Tetanus, diphtheria; tetanus, diphtheria and acellular pertussis[12]	7 years[12]	4 weeks	4 weeks if first dose of DTaP/DT was administered before the 1st birthday. 6 months (as final dose) if first dose of DTaP/DT or Tdap/Td was administered at or after the 1st birthday.	6 months if first dose of DTaP/DT was administered before the 1st birthday.
Human papillomavirus[13]	9 years	Routine dosing intervals are recommended.[13]		
Hepatitis A[10]	N/A	6 months		
Hepatitis B[1]	N/A	4 weeks	8 weeks **and** at least 16 weeks after first dose.	
Inactivated poliovirus[6]	N/A	4 weeks	4 weeks[6]	6 months[6]
Measles, mumps, rubella[8]	N/A	4 weeks		
Varicella[9]	N/A	3 months if younger than age 13 years. 4 weeks if age 13 years or older.		

NOTE: The above recommendations must be read along with the footnotes of this schedule (Figure 3).

Figure 2 Continued

For further guidance on the use of the vaccines mentioned below, see: http://www.cdc.gov/vaccines/hcp/acip-recs/index.html.
For vaccine recommendations for persons 19 years of age and older, see the Adult Immunization Schedule.

Additional Information

- For contraindications and precautions to use of a vaccine and for additional information regarding that vaccine, vaccination providers should consult the relevant ACIP statement available online at http://www.cdc.gov/vaccines/hcp/acip-recs/index.html.
- For purposes of calculating intervals between doses, 4 weeks = 28 days. Intervals of 4 months or greater are determined by calendar months.
- Vaccine doses administered 4 days or less before the minimum interval are considered valid. Does of any vaccine administered ≥ 5 days earlier than the minimum interval or minimum age should not be counted as valid doses and should be repeated as age-appropriate. The repeat dose should be spaced after the invalid dose by the recommended minimum interval. For further details, see *MMWR, General Recommendations on Immunization and Reports*/Vol. 60/No. 2;Table 1. *Recommended and minimum ages and intervals between vaccine doses* available online at http://www.cdc.gov/mmwr/pdf/rr/rr6002.pdf.
- Information on travel vaccine requirements and recommendations is available at http://wwwnc.cdc.gov/travel/destinations/list.
- For vaccination of persons with primary and secondary immunodeficiencies, see Table 13, *"Vaccination of persons with primary and secondary immunodeficiencies,"* in *General Recommendations on Immunization* (ACIP), available at http://www.cdc.gov/mmwr/pdf/rr/rr6002.pdf.; and American Academy of Pediatrics, "Immunization in Special Clinical Circumstances," in Kimberlin DW, Brady MT, Jackson MA, Long SS eds. *Red Book: 2015 report of the Committee on Infectious Diseases. 30th ed.* Elk Grove Village, IL: American Academy of Pediatrics.

1. Hepatitis B (HepB) vaccine. (Minimum age: birth)

Routine vaccination:

At birth:

- Administer monovalent HepB vaccine to all newborns before hospital discharge.
- For infants born to hepatitis B surface antigen (HBsAg)-positive mothers, administer HepB vaccine and 0.5 mL of hepatitis B immune globulin (HBIG) within 12 hours of birth. These infants should be tested for HBsAg and antibody to HBsAg (anti-HBs) at age 9 through 18 months (preferably at the next well-child visit) or 1 to 2 months after completion of the HepB series if the series was delayed; CDC recently recommend testing occur at age 9 through 12 months; see http://www.cdc.gov/mmwr/preview/mmwrhtml/mm6439a6.htm.
- If mother's HBsAg status is unknown, within 12 hours of birth administer HepB vaccine regardless of birth weight. For infants weighing less than 2,000 grams, administer HBIG in addition to HepB vaccine within 12 hours of birth. Determine mother's HBsAg status as soon as possible and, if mother is HBsAg-positive, also administer HBIG for infants weighing 2,000 grams or more as soon as possible, but no later than age 7 days.

Figure 3 Footnotes: Recommended immunization schedule for persons aged 0 through 18 years in the United States, 2016

Doses following the birth dose:

- The second dose should be administered at age 1 or 2 months. Monovalent HepB vaccine should be used for doses administered before age 6 weeks.

- Infants who did not receive a birth dose should receive 3 doses of a HepB-containing vaccine on a schedule of 0, 1 to 2 months, and 6 months starting as soon as feasible. See Figure 2.

- Administer the second dose 1 to 2 months after the first dose (minimum interval of 4 weeks), administer the third dose at least 8 weeks after the second dose AND at least 16 weeks after the **first** dose. The final (third or fourth) dose in the HepB vaccine series should be administered **no earlier than age 24 weeks.**

- Administration of a total of 4 doses of HepB vaccine is permitted when a combination vaccine containing HepB administered after the birth dose.

Catch-up vaccination:

- Unvaccinated persons should complete a 3-dose series.

- A 2-dose series (doses separated by at least 4 months) of adult formulation Recombivax HB is licensed for use in children aged 11 through 15 years.

- For other catch-up guidance, see Figure 2.

2. Rotavirus (RV) vaccines. (Minimum age: 6 weeks for both RV1 [Rotarix] and RV5 [RotaTeq])

Routine vaccination:

Administer a series of RV vaccine to all infants as follows:

1. If Rotarix is used, administer a 2-dose series at 2 and 4 months of age.
2. If RotaTeq is used, administer a 3-dose series at ages 2, 4, and 6 months.
3. If any dose in the series was RotaTeq or vaccine product is unknown for any dose in the series, a total of 3 doses of RV vaccine should be administered.

Catch-up vaccination:

- The maximum age for the first dose in the series is 14 weeks, 6 days; vaccination should not be initiated for infants aged 15 weeks, 0 days or older.

- The maximum age for the final dose in the series is 8 months, 0 days.

- For other catch-up guidance, see Figure 2.

3. Diphtheria and tetanus toxoids and acellular pertussis (DTaP) vaccine. (Minimum age: 6 weeks. Exception: DTaP-IPV [Kinrix, Quadracel]: 4 years)

Routine vaccination:

- Administer a 5-dose series of DTaP vaccine at ages 2, 4, 6, 15 through 18 months, and 4 through 6 years. The fourth dose may be administered as early as age 12 months, provided at least 6 months have elapsed since the third dose.

Figure 3 Continued

- Inadvertent administration of 4th DTaP dose early; If the fourth dose of DTaP was administered at least 4 months, but less than 6 months, after the third dose of DTaP, it need not be repeated.

Catch–up vaccination:
- The fifth dose of DTaP vaccine is not necessary if the fourth dose was administered at age 4 years or older.
- For other catch-up guidance, see Figure 2.

4. *Haemophilus influenzae* type b (Hib) conjugate vaccine. (Minimum age: 6 weeks for PRP-T [AC-THIB, DTaP-IPV/ Hib (Pentacel) and Hib-MenCY MenHibrix)], PRP-OMP [PedvaxHIB or COMVAX], 12 months for PRP-T [Hiberix])

Routine vaccination:
- Administer a 2- or 3-dose Hib vaccine primary series and a booster dose (dose 3 or 4 depending on vaccine used in primary series) at age 12 through 15 months to complete a full Hib vaccine series.
- The primary series with ActHIB, MenHibrix, or Pentacel consists of 3 doses and should be administered at 2, 4, and 6 months of age. The primary series with PedvaxHib or COMVAX consists of 2 doses and should be administered at 2 and 4 months of age; a dose at age 6 months is not indicated.
- One booster dose (dose 3 or 4 depending on vaccine used in primary series) of any Hib vaccine should be administered at age 12 through 15 months. An exception is Hiberix vaccine. Hiberix should only be used for the booster (final) dose in children aged 12 months through 4 years who have received at least 1 prior dose of Hib-containing vaccine.
- For recommendations on the use of MenHibrix in patients at increased risk for meningococcal disease, please refer to the meningococcal vaccine footnotes and also to *MMWR* February 28, 2014 / 63(RR01);1-13, available at http://www.cdc.gov/mmwr/PDF/ rr/rr6301.pdf.

Catch-up vaccination:
- If dose 1 was administered at ages 12 through 14 months, administer a second (final) dose at least 8 weeks after dose 1, regardless of Hib vaccine used in the primary series.
- If both doses were PRP-OMP (PedvaxHIB or COMVAX), and were administered before the first birthday, the third (and final) dose should be administered at age 12 through 59 months and at least 8 weeks after the second dose.
- If the first dose was administered at age 7 through 11 months, administer the second dose at least 4 weeks later and a third (and final) dose at age 12 through 15 months or 8 weeks after second dose, whichever is later.
- If first dose is administered before the first birthday and second dose administered at younger than 15 months, a third (and final) dose should be administered 8 weeks later.
- For unvaccinated children aged 15 months or older, administer only 1 dose.
- For other catch-up guidance, see Figure 2. For catch-up guidance related to MenHibrix, please see the meningococcal vaccine footnotes and also *MMWR* February 28, 2014 / 63(RR01);1-13, available at http://www.cdc.gov/mmwr/PDF/rr/rr6301.pdf.

Vaccination of persons with high-risk conditions:

- Children aged 12 through 59 months who are at increased risk for Hib disease, including chemotherapy recipients and those with anatomic or functional asplenia (including sickle cell disease), human immunodeficiency virus (HIV) infection, immunoglobulin deficiency, or early component complement deficiency, who have received either no doses or only 1 dose of Hib vaccine before 12 months of age, should receive 2 additional doses of Hib vaccine 8 weeks apart; children who received 2 or more doses of Hib vaccine before 12 months of age should receive 1 additional dose.

- For patients younger than 5 years of age undergoing chemotherapy or radiation treatment who received a Hib vaccine dose(s) within 14 days of starting therapy or during therapy, repeat the dose(s) at least 3 months following therapy completion.

- Recipients of hematopoietic stem cell transplant (HSCT) should be revaccinated with a 3-dose regimen of Hib vaccine starting 6 to 12 months after successful transplant, regardless of vaccination history; doses should be administered at least 4 weeks apart.

- A single dose of any Hib-containing vaccine should be administered to unimmunized* children and adolescents 15 months of age and older undergoing an elective splenectomy; if possible, vaccine should be administered at least 14 days before procedure.

- Hib vaccine is not routinely recommended for patients 5 years or older. However, 1 dose of Hib vaccine should be administered to unimmunized* persons aged 5 years or older who have anatomic or functional asplenia (including sickle cell disease) and unvaccinated persons 5 through 18 years of age with HIV infection.

  Patients who have not received a primary series and booster dose or at least 1 dose of Hib vaccine after 14 months of age are considered unimmunized.

5. Pneumococcal vaccines. (Minimum age: 6 weeks for PCV13, 2 years for PPSV23)

Routine vaccination with PCV13:

- Administer a 4-dose series of PCV13 vaccine at ages 2, 4, and 6 months and at age 12 through 15 months.
- For children aged 14 through 59 months who have received an age-appropriate series of 7-valent PCV (PCV7), administer a single supplemental dose of 13-valent PCV (PCV13).

Catch-up vaccination with PCV13:

- Administer 1 dose of PCV13 to all healthy children aged 24 through 59 months who are not completely vaccinated for their age.
- For other catch-up guidance, see Figure 2.

Vaccination of persons with high-risk conditions with PCV13 and PPSV23:

- All recommended PCV13 doses should be administered prior to PPSV23 vaccination if possible.
- For children 2 through 5 years of age with any of the following conditions: chronic heart disease (particularly cyanotic congenital heart disease and cardiac failure); chronic lung disease (including asthma if treated with high-dose oral corticosteroid therapy); diabetes mellitus; cerebrospinal fluid leak; cochlear implant; sickle cell disease and other hemoglobinopathies; anatomic or functional asplenia; HIV infection; chronic renal failure; nephrotic syndrome; diseases associated with treatment with immunosuppressive

Figure 3 Continued

31

drugs or radiation therapy, including malignant neoplasms, leukemias, lymphomas, and Hodgkin disease; solid organ transplantation; or congenital immunodeficiency:

1. Administer 1 dose of PCV13 if any incomplete schedule of 3 doses of PCV (PCV7 and/or PCV13) were received previously.
2. Administer 2 doses of PCV13 at least 8 weeks apart if unvaccinated or any incomplete schedule of fewer than 3 doses of PCV (PCV7 and/or PCV13) were received previously.
3. Administer 1 supplemental dose of PCV13 if 4 doses of PCV7 or other age-appropriate complete PCV7 series was received previously.
4. The minimum interval between doses of PCV (PCV7 or PCV13) is 8 weeks.
5. For children with no history of PPSV23 vaccination, administer PPSV23 at least 8 weeks after the most recent dose of PCV13.

- For children aged 6 through 18 years who have cerebrospinal fluid leak; cochlear implant; sickle cell disease and other hemoglobinopathies; anatomic or functional asplenia; congenital or acquired immunodeficiencies; HIV infection; chronic renal failure; nephrotic syndrome; diseases associated with treatment with immunosuppressive drugs or radiation therapy, including malignant neoplasms, leukemias, lymphomas, and Hodgkin disease; generalized malignancy; solid organ transplantation; or multiple myeloma:

1. If neither PCV13 nor PPSV23 has been received previously, administer 1 dose of PCV13 now and 1 dose of PPSV23 at least 8 weeks later.
2. If PCV13 has been received previously but PPSV23 has not, administer 1 dose of PPSV23 at least 8 weeks after the most recent dose of PCV13.
3. If PPSV23 has been received but PCV13 has not, administer 1 dose of PCV13 at least 8 weeks after the most recent dose of PPSV23.

- For children aged 6 through 18 years with chronic heart disease (particularly cyanotic congenital heart disease and cardiac failure), chronic lung disease (including asthma if treated with high-dose oral corticosteroid therapy), diabetes mellitus, alcoholism, or chronic liver disease, who have not received PPSV23, administer 1 dose of PPSV23. If PCV13 has been received previously, then PPSV23 should be administered at least 8 weeks after any prior PCV13 dose.

- A single revaccination with PPSV23 should be administered 5 years after the first dose to children with sickle cell disease or other hemoglobinopathies; anatomic or functional asplenia; congenital or acquired immunodeficiencies; HIV infection; chronic renal failure; nephrotic syndrome; diseases associated with treatment with immunosuppressive drugs or radiation therapy, including malignant neoplasms, leukemias, lymphomas, and Hodgkin disease; generalized malignancy; solid organ transplantation; or multiple myeloma.

6. Inactivated poliovirus vaccine (IPV). (Minimum age: 6 weeks)

Routine vaccination:

- Administer a 4-dose series of IPV at ages 2, 4, 6 through 18 months, and 4 through 6 years. The final dose in the series should be administered on or after the fourth birthday and at least 6 months after the previous dose.

Catch-up vaccination:

- In the first 6 months of life, minimum age and minimum intervals are only recommended if the person is at risk of imminent exposure to circulating poliovirus (i.e., travel to a polio-endemic region or during an outbreak).
- If 4 or more doses are administered before age 4 years, an additional dose should be administered at age 4 through 6 years and at least 6 months after the previous dose.
- A fourth dose is not necessary if the third dose was administered at age 4 years or older and at least 6 months after the previous dose.
- If both OPV and IPV were administered as part of a series, a total of 4 doses should be administered, regardless of the child's current age. If only OPV were administered, and all doses were given prior to 4 years of age, one dose of IPV should be given at 4 years or older, at least 4 weeks after the last OPV dose.
- IPV is not routinely recommended for U.S. residents aged 18 years or older.
- For other catch-up guidance, see Figure 2.

7. Influenza vaccines. (Minimum age: 6 months for inactivated influenza vaccine [IIV], 2 years for live, attenuated influenza vaccine [LAIV])

Routine vaccination:

- Administer influenza vaccine annually to all children beginning at age 6 months. For most healthy, nonpregnant persons aged 2 through 49 years, either LAIV or IIV may be used. However, LAIV should NOT be administered to some persons, including 1) persons who have experienced severe allergic reactions to LAIV, any of its components, or to a previous dose of ay other influenza vaccine; 2) children 2 through 17 years receiving aspirin or aspirin-containing products; 3) persons who are allergic to eggs; 4) pregnant women; 5) immunosuppressed persons; 6) children 2 through 4 years of age with asthma or who had wheezing in the past 12 months; or 7) persons who have taken influenza antiviral medications in the previous 48 hours. For all other contraindications and precautions to use of LAIV, see *MMWR* August 7, 2015 / 64(30):818-25 available at http://www.cdc.gov/mmwr/pdf/wk/mm6430.pdf.

For children aged 6 months through 8 years:

- For the 2015–16 season, administer 2 doses (separated by at least 4 weeks) to children who are receiving influenza vaccine for the first time. Some children in this age group who have been vaccinated previously will also need 2 doses. For additional guidance,

Figure 3 Continued

follow dosing guidelines in the 2015–16 ACIP influenza vaccine recommendations, *MMWR* August 7, 2015 / 64(30):818-25, available at http://www.cdc.gov/mmwr/pdf/wk/mm6430.pdf.

- For the 2016–17 season, follow dosing guidelines in the 2016 ACIP influenza vaccine recommendations.

For persons aged 9 years and older:
- Administer 1 dose.

8. **Measles, mumps, and rubella (MMR) vaccine. (Minimum age: 12 months for routine vaccination)**
   Routine vaccination:
   - Administer a 2-dose series of MMR vaccine at ages 12 through 15 months and 4 through 6 years. The second dose may be administered before age 4 years, provided at least 4 weeks have elapsed since the first dose.
   - Administer 1 dose of MMR vaccine to infants aged 6 through 11 months before departure from the United States for international travel. These children should be revaccinated with 2 doses of MMR vaccine, the first at age 12 through 15 months (12 months if the child remains in an area where disease risk is high), and the second dose at least 4 weeks later.
   - Administer 2 doses of MMR vaccine to children aged 12 months and older before departure from the United States for international travel. The first dose should be administered on or after age 12 months and the second dose at least 4 weeks later.

   Catch-up vaccination:
   - Ensure that all school-aged children and adolescents have had 2 doses of MMR vaccine; the minimum interval between the 2 doses is 4 weeks.

9. **Varicella (VAR) vaccine. (Minimum age: 12 months)**
   Routine vaccination:
   - Administer a 2-doses series of VAR vaccine at ages 12 through 15 months and 4 through 6 years. The second dose may be administered before age 4 years, provided at least 3 months have elapsed since the first dose. If the second dose was administered at least 4 weeks after the first dose, it can be accepted as valid.

   Catch-up vaccination:
   - Ensure that all persons aged 7 through 18 years without evidence of immunity (see *MMWR* 2007 / 56 [No. RR-4], available at http://www.cdc.gov/mmwr/pdf/rr/rr5604.pdf) have 2 doses of varicella vaccine. For children aged 7 through 12 years, the recommended minimum interval between doses is 3 months (if the second dose was administered at least 4 weeks after the first dose, it can be accepted as valid); for persons aged 13 years and older, the minimum interval between doses is 4 weeks.

10. **Hepatitis A (HepA) vaccine. (Minimum age: 12 months)**
    Routine vaccination:
    - Initiate the 2-dose HepA vaccine series at 12 through 23 months; separate the 2 doses by 6 to 18 months.
    - Children who have received 1 dose of HepA vaccine before age 24 months should receive a second dose 6 to 18 months after the first dose.

- For any person aged 2 years and older who has not already received the HepA vaccine series, 2 doses of HepA vaccine separated by 6 to 18 months may be administered if immunity against hepatitis A virus infection is desired.

Catch-up vaccination:
- The minimum interval between the 2 doses is 6 months.

Special populations:
- Administer 2 doses of HepA vaccine at least 6 months apart to previously unvaccinated persons who live in areas where vaccination programs target older children, or who are at increased risk for infection. This includes persons traveling to or working in countries that have high or intermediate endemicity of infection; men having sex with men; users of injection and non-injection illicit drugs; persons who work with HAV-infected primates or with HAV in a research laboratory; persons with clotting-factor disorders; persons with chronic liver disease; and persons who anticipate close personal contact (e.g., household or regular babysitting) with an international adoptee during the first 60 days after arrival in the United States from a country with high or intermediate endemicity. The first dose should be administered as soon as the adoption is planned, ideally 2 or more weeks before the arrival of the adoptee.

11. **Meningococcal vaccines. (Minimum age: 6 weeks for Hib-MenCY [MenHibrix], 9 months for MenACWY-D [Menactra], 2 months for MenACWY-CRM [Menveo], 10 years for serogroup B meningococcal [MenB] vaccines: MenB-4C [Bexsero] and MenB-FHbp [Trumenba])**

Routine vaccination:
- Administer a single dose of Menactra or Menveo vaccine at age 11 through 12 years, with a booster dose at age 16 years.
- Adolescents aged 11 through 18 years with human immunodeficiency virus (HIV) infection should receive a 2-dose primary series of Menactra or Menveo with at least 8 weeks between doses.
- For children aged 2 months through 18 years with high-risk conditions, see below.

Catch-up vaccination:
- Administer Menactra or Menveo vaccine at age 13 through 18 years if not previously vaccinated.
- If the first dose is administered at age 13 through 15 years, a booster dose should be administered at age 16 through 18 years with a minimum interval of at least 8 weeks between doses.
- If the first dose is administered at age 16 years or older, a booster dose is not needed.
- For other catch-up guidance, see Figure 2.

Clinical discretion:
- Young adults aged 16 through 23 years (preferred age range is 16 through 18 years) may be vaccinated with either a 2-dose series of Bexsero or a 3-dose series of Trumenba vaccine to provide short-term protection against most strains of serogroup B meningococcal disease. The two MenB vaccines are not interchangeable; the same vaccine product must be used for all doses.

Figure 3 Continued

Vaccination of persons with high-risk conditions and other persons at increased risk of disease:

Children with anatomic or functional asplenia (including sickle cell disease):

Meningococcal conjugate ACWY vaccines:

1. Menveo
   - *Children who initiate vaccination at 8 weeks:* Administer doses at 2, 4, 6, and 12 months of age.
   - *Unvaccinated children who initiate vaccination at 7 through 23 months:* Administer 2 doses, with the second dose at least 12 weeks after the first dose AND after the first birthday.
   - *Children 24 months and older who have not received a complete series:* Administer 2 primary doses at least 8 weeks apart.

2. MenHibrix
   - *Children who initiate vaccination at 6 weeks:* Administer doses at 2, 4, 6, and 12 through 15 months of age.
   - If the first dose of MenHibrix is given at or after 12 months of age, a total of 2 doses should be given at least 8 weeks apart to ensure protection against serogroups C and Y meningococcal disease.

3. Menactra
   - *Children 24 months and older who have not received a complete series:* Administer 2 primary doses at least 8 weeks apart. If Menactra is administered to a child with asplenia (including sickle cell disease), do not administer Menactra until 2 years of age and at least 4 weeks after the completion of all PCV13 doses.

Meningococcal B vaccines:

1. Bexsero or Trumenba
   - *Persons 10 years or older who have not received a complete series.* Administer a 2-dose series of Bexsero, at least 1 month apart. Or a 3-dose series of Trumenba, with the second dose at least 2 months after the first and the third dose at least 6 months after the first. The two MenB vaccines are not interchangeable; the same vaccine product must be used for all doses.

Children with persistent complement component deficiency (includes persons with inherited or chronic deficiencies in C3, C5-9, properidin, factor D, factor H, or taking eculizumab (Soliris®):

Meningococcal conjugate ACWY vaccines:

1. Menveo
   - *Children who initiate vaccination at 8 weeks:* Administer doses at 2, 4, 6, and 12 months of age.
   - *Unvaccinated children who initiate vaccination at 7 through 23 months:* Administer 2 doses, with the second dose at least 12 weeks after the first dose AND after the first birthday.
   - *Children 24 months and older who have not received a complete series:* Administer 2 primary doses at least 8 weeks apart.

2. MenHibrix
- *Children who initiate vaccination 6 weeks:* Administer doses at 2, 4, 6, and 12 through 15 months of age.
  - If the first dose of MenHibrix is given at or after 12 months of age, a total of 2 doses should be given at least 8 weeks apart to ensure protection against serogroups C and Y meningococcal disease.
3. Menactra
- *Children 9 through 23 months:* Administer 2 primary doses at least 12 weeks apart.
- *Children 24 months and older who have not received a complete series:* Administer 2 primary doses at least 8 weeks apart.

Meningococcal B vaccines:
1. Bexsero or Trumenba
- *Persons 10 years or older who have not received a complete series.* Administer a 2-dose series of Bexsero, at least 1 month apart. Or a 3-dose series of Trumenba, with the second dose at least 2 months after the first and the third dose at least 6 months after the first. The two MenB vaccines are not interchangeable; the same vaccine product must be used for all doses.

For children who travel to or reside in countries in which meningococcal disease is hyperendemic or epidemic, including countries in the African meningitis belt or the Hajj
- administer an age-appropriate formulation and series of Menactra or Menveo for protection against serogroups A and W meningococcal disease. Prior receipt of MenHibrix is not sufficient for children traveling to the meningitis belt or the Hajj because it does not contain serogroups A or W.

For children at risk during a community outbreak attributable to a vaccine serogroup
- administer or complete an age- and formulation-appropriate series of MenHibrix, Menactra, or Menveo, Bexsero or Trumenba.

For booster doses among persons with high-risk conditions, refer to *MMWR* 2013 / 62(RR02);1-22, available at http://www.cdc.gov/mmwr/preview/mmwrhtml/rr6202a1.htm.

For other catch-up recommendations for these persons, and complete information on use of meningococcal vaccines, including guidance related to vaccination of persons at increased risk of infection, see *MMWR* March 22, 2013 / 62(RR02);1-22, and *MMWR* October 23, 2015 / 64(41); 1171-1176 available at http://www.cdc.gov/mmwr/pdf/rr/rr6202pdf, and http://www.cdc.gov/mmwr/pdf/wk/mm6441.pdf.

12. Tetanus and diphtheria toxoids and acellular pertussis (Tdap) vaccine. (Minimum age: 10 years for both Boostrix and Adacel)
Routine vaccination:
- Administer 1 dose of Tdap vaccine to all adolescents aged 11 through 12 years.
- Tdap may be administered regardless of the interval since the last tetanus and diphtheria toxoid-containing vaccine.

Figure 3 Continued

- Administer 1 dose of Tdap vaccine to pregnant adolescents during each pregnancy (preferred during 27 through 36 weeks gestation) regardless of time since prior Td or Tdap vaccination.

Catch-up vaccination:
- Persons aged 7 years and older who are not fully immunized with DTaP vaccine should receive Tdap vaccine as 1 (preferably the first) dose in the catch-up series; if additional doses are needed, use Td vaccine. For children 7 through 10 years who receive a dose of Tdap as part of the catch-up series, an adolescent Tdap vaccine dose at age 11 through 12 years should NOT be administered. Td should be administered instead 10 years after the Tdap dose.
- Persons aged 11 through 18 years who have not received Tdap vaccine should receive a dose followed by tetanus and diphtheria toxoids (Td) booster doses every 10 years thereafter.
- Inadvertent doses of DTaP vaccine:
  - If administered inadvertently to a child aged 7 through 10 years may count as part of the catch-up series. This dose may count as the adolescent Tdap dose, or the child can later receive a Tdap booster dose at age 11 through 12 years.
  - If administered inadvertently to an adolescent aged 11 through 18 years, the dose should be counted as the adolescent Tdap booster.
  - For other catch-up guidance, see Figure 2.

13. **Human papillomavirus (HPV) vaccines. (Minimum age: 9 years for 2vHPV [Cervarix], 4vHPV [Gardasil] and 9vHPV [Gardasil 9])**

Routine vaccination:
- Administer a 3-dose series of HPV vaccine on a schedule of 0, 1–2, and 6 months to all adolescents aged 11 through 12 years. 9vHPV, 4vHPV or 2vHPV may be used for females, and only 9vHPV or 4vHPV may be used for males.
- The vaccine series may be started at age 9 years.
- Administer the second dose 1 to 2 months after the first dose (minimum interval of 4 weeks); administer the third dose 16 weeks after the second dose (minimum interval of 12 weeks) and 24 weeks after the first dose.
- Administer HPV vaccine beginning at age 9 years to children and youth with any history of sexual abuse or assault who have not initiated or completed the 3-dose series.

Catch-up vaccination:
- Administer the vaccine series to females (2vHPV or 4vHPV or 9vHPV) and males (4vHPV or 9vHPV) at age 13 through 18 years if not previously vaccinated.
- Use recommended routine dosing intervals (see Routine vaccination above) for vaccine series catch-up.

Figure 3 Continued

2016 ADULT IMMUNIZATION SCHEDULES

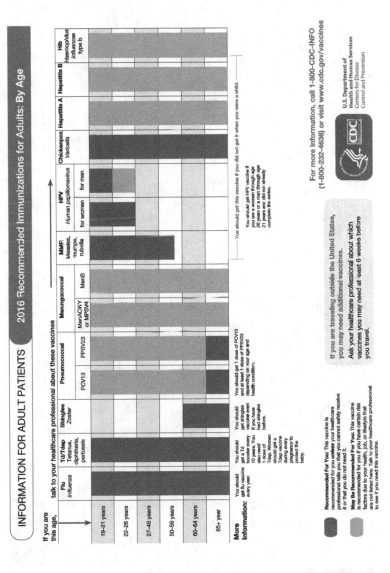

Figure 4 2016 recommended adult immunization schedules

VACCINE ▼ INDICATION ▶	Pregnancy	Immunocompromising conditions (excluding HIV infection) 4,6,7,8,13	HIV Infection CD4+ count (cells/μL) 4,6,7,8,13 <200	HIV Infection CD4+ count ≥200	Men who have sex with men (MSM)	Kidney failure, end-stage renal disease, on hemodialysis	Heart disease, chronic lung disease, chronic alcoholism	Asplenia and persistent complement component deficiencies 6,11,12	Chronic liver disease	Diabetes	Healthcare personnel
Influenza*,2	1 dose annually										
Tetanus, diphtheria, pertussis (Td/Tdap)*,3	1 dose Tdap each pregnancy	Substitute Tdap for Td once, then Td booster every 10 yrs									
Varicella*,4	Contraindicated	Contraindicated	Contraindicated	2 doses							
Human papillomavirus (HPV) Female*,5		3 doses through age 26 yrs	3 doses through age 26 yrs		3 doses through age 26 yrs						
Human papillomavirus (HPV) Male*,5		3 doses through age 26 yrs	3 doses through age 26 yrs		3 doses through age 21 yrs						
Zoster*,6	Contraindicated	Contraindicated	Contraindicated		1 dose						
Measles, mumps, rubella (MMR)*,7	Contraindicated	Contraindicated	Contraindicated	1 or 2 doses depending on indication							
Pneumococcal 13-valent conjugate (PCV13)*,8						1 dose					
Pneumococcal polysaccharide (PPSV23)*,8						1, 2, or 3 doses depending on indication					
Hepatitis A*,9						2 or 3 doses depending on vaccine					
Hepatitis B*,10						3 doses					
Meningococcal 4-valent conjugate (MenACWY) or polysaccharide (MPSV4)*,11						1 or more doses depending on indication					
Meningococcal B (MenB)*,11						2 or 3 doses depending on vaccine					
Haemophilus influenzae type b (Hib)*,12		3 doses post-HSCT recipients only				1 dose					

*Covered by the Vaccine Injury Compensation Program

Recommended for all persons who meet the age requirement, lack documentation of vaccination, or lack evidence of past infection; zoster vaccine is recommended regardless of past episode of zoster

Recommended for persons with a risk factor (medical, occupational, lifestyle, or other indication)

No recommendation

Contraindicated

U.S. Department of Health and Human Services
Centers for Disease Control and Prevention

CDC

These schedules indicate the recommended age groups and medical indications for which administration of currently licensed vaccines is commonly recommended for adults aged ≥19 years, as of February 2016. For all vaccines being recommended on the Adult Immunization Schedule: a vaccine series does not need to be restarted, regardless of the time that has elapsed between doses. Licensed combination vaccines may be used whenever any components of the combination are indicated and when the vaccine's other components are not contraindicated. For detailed recommendations on all vaccines, including those used primarily for travelers or those issued during the year, consult the manufacturers' package inserts and the complete statements from the Advisory Committee on Immunization Practices (www.cdc.gov/vaccines/hcp/acip-recs/index.html). Use of trade names and commercial sources is for identification only and does not imply endorsement by the U.S. Department of Health and Human Services.

Figure 5 Vaccines that might be indicated for adults aged 19 years or older based on medical and other indications

1. Additional information

- Additional guidance for the use of the vaccines described in this supplement is available at www.cdc.gov/vaccines/hcp/acip-recs/index.html.
- Information on vaccination recommendations when vaccination status is unknown and other general immunization information can be found in the General Recommendations on Immunization at www.cdc.gov/mmwr/preview/mmwrhtml/rr6002a1.htm.
- Information on travel vaccine requirements and recommendations (e.g., for hepatitis A and B, meningococcal, and other vaccines) is available at www.cdc.gov/travel/destinations/list.
- Additional information and resources regarding vaccination of pregnant women can be found at www.cdc.gov/vaccines/adults/rec-vac/pregnant.html.

2. Influenza vaccination

- Annual vaccination against influenza is recommended for all persons aged ≥6 months. A list of currently available influenza vaccines can be found at http://www.cdc.gov/flu/protect/vaccine/vaccines.htm.
- Persons aged ≥6 months, including pregnant women, can receive the inactivated influenza vaccine (IIV). An age-appropriate IIV formulation should be used.
- Intradermal IIV is an option for persons aged 18 through 64 years.
- High-dose IIV is an option for persons aged ≥65 years.
- Live attenuated influenza vaccine (LAIV [FluMist]) is an option for healthy, non-pregnant persons aged 2 through 49 years.
- Recombinant influenza vaccine (RIV [Flublok]) is approved for persons aged ≥18 years.
- RIV, which does not contain any egg protein, may be administered to persons aged ≥18 years with egg allergy of any severity; IIV may be used with additional safety measures for persons with hives-only allergy to eggs.
- Health care personnel who care for severely immunocompromised persons who require care in a protected environment should receive IIV or RIV; health care personnel who receive LAIV should avoid providing care for severely immunosuppressed persons for 7 days after vaccination.

3. Tetanus, diphtheria, and acellular pertussis (Td/Tdap) vaccination

- Administer 1 dose of Tdap vaccine to pregnant women during each pregnancy (preferably during 27–36 weeks' gestation) regardless of interval since prior Td or Tdap vaccination.
- Persons aged ≥11 years who have not received Tdap vaccine or for whom vaccine status is unknown should receive a dose of Tdap followed by tetanus and diphtheria toxoids (Td) booster doses every 10 years thereafter. Tdap can be administered regardless of interval since the most recent tetanus or diphtheria-toxoid-containing vaccine.
- Adults with an unknown or incomplete history of completing a 3-dose primary vaccination series with Td-containing vaccines should begin or complete a primary vaccination series including a Tdap dose.
- For unvaccinated adults, administer the first 2 doses at least 4 weeks apart and the third dose 6–12 months after the second.

Figure 6 Footnotes: Recommended immunization schedule for adults aged 19 years or older, United States, 2016

- For incompletely vaccinated (i.e., less than 3 doses) adults, administer remaining doses.
- Refer to the ACIP statement for recommendations for administering Td/Tdap as prophylaxis in wound management (see footnote 1).

4. Varicella vaccination

- All adults without evidence of immunity to varicella (as defined below) should receive 2 doses of single-antigen varicella vaccine or a second dose if they have received only 1 dose.
- Vaccination should be emphasized for those who have close contact with persons at high risk for severe disease (e.g., health care personnel and family contacts of persons with immunocompromising conditions) or are at high risk for exposure or transmission (e.g., teachers; child care employees; residents and staff members of institutional settings, including correctional institutions; college students; military personnel; adolescents and adults living in households with children; nonpregnant women of childbearing age; and international travelers).
- Pregnant women should be assessed for evidence of varicella immunity. Women who do not have evidence of immunity should receive the first dose of varicella vaccine upon completion or termination of pregnancy and before discharge from the health care facility. The second dose should be administered 4–8 weeks after the first dose.
- Evidence of immunity to varicella in adults includes any of the following:
  - documentation of 2 doses of varicella vaccine at least 4 weeks apart;
  - U.S.-born before 1980, except health care personnel and pregnant women;
  - history of varicella based on diagnosis or verification of varicella disease by a health care provider;
  - history of herpes zoster based on diagnosis or verification of herpes zoster disease by a health care provider; or
  - laboratory evidence of immunity or laboratory confirmation of disease.

5. Human papillomavirus (HPV) vaccination

- Three HPV vaccines are licensed for use in females (bivalent HPV vaccine [2vHPV], quadrivalent HPV vaccine [4vHPV], and 9-valent HPV vaccine [9vHPV]) and two HPV vaccines are licensed for use in males (4vHPV and 9vHPV).
- For females, 2vHPV, 4vHPV, or 9vHPV is recommended in a 3-dose series for routine vaccination at age 11 or 12 years and for those aged 13 through 26 years, if not previously vaccinated.
- For males, 4vHPV or 9vHPV is recommended in a 3-dose series for routine vaccination at age 11 or 12 years and for those aged 13 through 21 years, if not previously vaccinated. Males aged 22 through 26 years may be vaccinated. HPV vaccination is recommended for men who have sex with men through age 26 years who did not get any or all doses when they were younger.
- Vaccination is recommended for immunocompromised persons (including those with HIV infection) through age 26 years who did not get any or all doses when they were younger.

- A complete HPV vaccination series consists of 3 doses. The second dose should be administered 4–8 weeks (minimum interval of 4 weeks) after the first dose; the third dose should be administered 24 weeks after the first dose and 16 weeks after the second dose (minimum interval of 12 weeks).
- HPV vaccines are not recommended for use in pregnant women. However, pregnancy testing is not needed before vaccination. If a woman is found to be pregnant after initiating the vaccination series, no intervention is needed; the remainder of the 3-doses series should be delayed until completion or termination of pregnancy.

6. Zoster vaccination

- A single dose of zoster vaccine is recommended for adults aged ≥60 years regardless of whether they report a prior episode of herpes zoster. Although the vaccine is licensed by the U.S. Food and Drun Administration for use among and can be administered to persons aged ≥50 years, ACIP recommends that vaccination begin at age 60 years.
- Persons aged ≥60 years with chronic medical conditions may be vaccinated unless their condition constitutes a contraindication, such a pregnancy or severe immunodeficiency.

7. Measles, mumps, rubella (MMR) vaccination

- Adults born before 1957 are generally considered immune to measles and mumps. All adults born in 1957 or later should have documentation of 1 or more doses of MMR vaccine uless they have a medical contraindication to the vaccine or laboratory evidence of immunity to each of the three diseases. Documentation of provided-diagnosed disease is not considered acceptable evidence of immunity for measles, mumps, or rubella.

Measles component:

- A routine second dose of MMR vaccine, administered a minimum of 28 days after the first dose, is recommended for adults who:
  — are students in postsecondary educational institutions,
  — work in a health care facility, or
  — plan to travel internationally.
- Persons who received inactivated (killed) measles vaccine or measles vaccine of unknown type during 1963–1967 should be revaccinated with 2 doses of MMR vaccine.

Mumps component:

- A routine second dose of MMR vaccine, administered a minimum of 28 days after the first dose, is recommended for adults who:
  — are students in a postsecondary educational institution,
  — work in a health care facility, or
  — plan to travel internationally.
- Persons vaccinated before 1979 with either killed mumps vaccine or mumps vaccine of unknown type who are at high risk for mumps infection (e.g., persons who are working in a health care facility) should be considered for revaccination with 2 doses of MMR vaccine.

Figure 6 Continued

43

Rubella component:

• For women of childbearing age, regardless of birth year, rubella immunity should be determined. If there is no evidence of immunity, women who are not pregnant should be vaccinated. Pregnant women who do not have evidence of immunity should receive MMR vaccine upon completion or termination of pregnancy and before discharge from health care facility.

Health care personnel born before 1957:

• For unvaccinated health care personnel born before 1957 who lack laboratory evidence of measles, mumps, and/or rubell immunity or laboratory confirmation of disease, health care facilities should consider vaccinating personnel with 2 doses of MMR vaccine at the appropriate interval for measles and mumps or 1 dose of MMR vaccine for rubella.

8. Pneumococcal vaccination

• General information

   — Adults are recommend to receive 1 dose of 13-valent pneumococcal conjugate vaccine (PCV13) and 1, 2, or 3 doses (depending on indication) of 23-valent pneumococcal polysaccharide vaccine (PPSV23).

   — PCV13 should be administered at least 1 year after PPSV23.

   — PPSV23 should be administered at least 1 year after PCV13, except among adults with immunocompromising conditions, anatomical or functional asplenia, cerebrospinal fluid leak, or cochlear implant, for whom the interval should be at least 8 weeks, the interval between PPSV23 does should be at least 5 years.

   — No additional dose of PPSV23 is indicated for adults vaccinated with PPSV23 at age ≥65 years.

   — When both PCV13 and PPSV23 are indicated, PCV13 should be administered first; PCV13 and PPSV23 should not be administered during the same visit.

   — When indicated, PCV13 and PPSV23 should be administered to adults whose pneumococcal vaccination history is incomplete or unknown.

• Adults aged ≥65 years (immunocompetent) who:

   — have not received PCV13 or PPSV23; administer PCV13 followed by PPSV23 at least 1 year after PCV13.

   — have not received PCV13 but have received a dose of PPSV23 at age ≥65 years; administer PCV13 at least 1 year after PPSV23.

   — have not received PCV13 but have received 1 or more doses of PPSV23 at age <65 years; administer PCV13 at least 1 year after the most recent dose of PPSV23. Administer a dose of PPSV23 at least 1 year after PCV13 and at least 5 years after the most recent dose of PPSV23.

   — have received PCV13 but not PPSV23 at age <65 years: administer PPSV23 at least 1 year after PCV13.

   — have received PCV13 and 1 or more doses of PPSV23 at age <65 years: administer PPSV23 at least 1 year after PCV13 and at least 5 years after the most recent dose of PPSV23.

- Adults aged ≥19 years with immunocompromising conditions or anatomical or functional asplenia (defined below) who:
  - have not received PCV13 or PPSV23: administer PCV13 followed by PPSV23 at least 8 weeks after PCV13. Administer a second dose of PPSV23 at least 5 years after the first dose of PPSV23.
  - have not received PCV13 but have received 1 dose of PPSV23; administer PCV13 at least 1 year after the PPSV23. Administer a second dose of PPSV23 at least 8 weeks after PCV13 and at least 5 years after the first dose of PPSV23.
  - have not received PCV13 but have received 2 doses of PPSV23; administer PCV13 at least 1 year after the most recent dose of PPSV23.
  - have received PCV13 but not PPSV23; administer PPSV23 at least 8 weeks after PCV13. Administer a second dose of PPSV23 at least 5 years after the first dose of PPSV23.
  - have received PCV13 and 1 dose of PPSV23: administer a second dose of PPSV23 at least 8 weeks after PCV13 and at least 5 years after the first dose of PPSV23.
  - If the most recent dose of PPSV23 was administered at age <65 years, at age ≥65 years, administer a dose of PPSV23 at least 8 weeks after PCV13 and at least 5 years after the last dose of PPSV23.
  - Immunocompromising conditions that are indications for pneumococcal vaccination are: congenital or acquired immuno-deficiency (including B- or T-lymphocyte deficiency, complement deficiencies, and phagocytic disorders excluding chronic granulomatous disease), HIV infection, chronic renal failure, nephrotic syndrome, leukemia, lymphoma, Hodgkin disease, generalized malignancy, multiple myeloma, solid organ transplant, and iatrogenic immunosuppression (including long-term systemic corticosteroids and radiation therapy).
  - Anatomical or functional asplenia that are indications for pneumococcal vaccination are; sickle cell disease and other hemo-globinopathies, congenital or acquired asplenia, splenic dysfunction, and splenectomy. Administer pneumococcal vaccines at least 2 weeks before immunosuppressive therapy or an elective splenectomy, and as soon as possible to adults who are newly diagnosed with asymptomatic or symptomatic HIV infection.
- Adults aged ≥19 years with cerebrospinal fluid leaks or cochlear implants: administer PCV13 followed by PPSV23 at least 8 weeks after PCV13; no additional dose of PPSV23 is indicated if aged <65 years. If PPSV23 was administered at age <65 years, at age ≥65 years, administer another dose of PPSV23 at least 5 years after the last dose of PPSV23.
- Adults aged 19 through 64 years with chronic heart disease (including congestive heart failure and cardiomyopathies, excluding hypertension), chronic lung disease (including chronic obstructive lung disease, emphysema, and asthma), chronic liver disease (including cirrhosis), alcoholism, or diabetes mellitus, or who smoke cigarettes; administer PPSV23. At age ≥65 years, administer PCV13 at least 1 year after PPSV23, followed by another dose of PPSV23 at least 1 year after PCV13 and at least 5 years after the last dose of PPSV23.
- Routine pneumococcal vaccination is not recommended for American Indian/Alaska Native or other adults unless they have an indica-tion as above; however, public health authorities may consider recommending the use of pneumococcal vaccines for American Indians/Alaska Natives or other adults who live in areas with increased risk for invasive pneumococcal disease.

Figure 6 Continued

45

9. Hepatitis A vaccination

- Vaccinate any person seeking protection from hepatitis A virus (HAV) infection and persons with any of the following indications:
  - men who have sex with men;
  - persons who use injection or noninjection illicit drugs;
  - persons working with HAV-infected primates or with HAV in a research laboratory setting;
  - persons with chronic liver disease and persons who receive clotting factor concentrates;
  - persons traveling to or working in countries that have high or intermediate endemicity of hepatitis A (see footnote 1); and
  - unvaccinated persons who anticipate close personal contact (e.g., household or regular babysitting) with an international adoptee during the first 60 days after arrival in the United Stated from a country with high or intermediate endemicity of hepatitis A (see footnote 1). The first dose of the 2-dose hepatitis A vaccine series should be administered as soon as adoption is planned, ideally 2 or more weeks before the arrival of the adoptee.
- Single-antigen vaccine formulations should be administered in a 2-dose schedule at either 0 and 6–12 months (Havrix), or 0 and 6–18 months (Vaqta). If the combined hepatitis A and hepatitis B vaccine (Twinrix) is used, administer 3 doses at 0, 1, and 6 months; alternatively, a 4-dose schedule may be used, administered on days 0, 7, and 21–30 followed by a booster dose at 12 months.

10. Hepatitis B vaccination

- Vaccinate any person seeking protection from hepatitis B virus (HBV) infection and persons with any of the following indications:
  - sexually active persons who are not in a long-term, mutually monogamous relationship (e.g., persons with more than 1 sex partner during the previous 6 months); persons seeking evaluation or treatment for a sexually transmitted disease (STD); current or recent injection drug users; and men who have sex with men;
  - health care personnel and public safety workers who are potentially exposed to blood or other infectious body fluids;
  - persons who are aged <60 years with diabetes as soon as feasible after diagnosis; persons with diabetes who are aged ≥60 years at the discretion of the treating clinician based on the likelihood of acquiring HBV infection, including the risk posed by an increased need for assisted blood glucose monitoring in long-term care facilities, the likelihood of experiencing chronic sequelae if infected with HBV, and the likelihood of immune response to vaccination;
  - persons with end-stage renal disease (including patients receiving hemodialysis), persons with HIV infection, and persons with chronic liver disease;
  - household contacts and sex partners of hepatitis B surface antigen-positive persons, clients and staff members of institutions for persons with developmental disabilities, and international travelers to regions with high or intermediate levels of endemic HBV infection (see footnote 1); and

— all adults in the following settings: STD treatment facilities, HIV testing and treatment facilities, factilities providing drug abuse treatment and prevention services, health care settings targeting services to injection drug users or men who have sex with men, correctional facilities, end-stage renal disease programs and facilities for chronic hemodialysis patients, and institutions and nonresidential day care facilities for persons with developmental disabilities.

• Administer missing doses to complete a 3-dose series of hepatitis B vaccine to those persons not vaccinated or not completely vaccinated. The second dose should be administered at least 1 month after the first dose; the third dose should be administered at least 2 months after the second dose (and at least 4 months after the first dose). If the combined hepatitis A and hepatitis B vaccine (Twinrix) is used, give 3 doses at 0, 1, and 6 months; alternatively, a 4-dose Twinrix schedule may be used, administered on days 0, 7, and 21–30, followed by a booster dose at 12 months.

• Adult patients receiving hemodialysis or with other immunocompromising conditions should receive 1 dose of 40 mcg/mL (Recombivax HB) administered on a 3-dose schedule at 0, 1, and 6 months or 2 doses of 20 mcg/mL (Engerix-B) administered simultaneously on a 4-dose schedule at 0, 1, 2, and 6 months.

11. Meningococcal vaccination

• General information
  — Serogroup A, C, W, and Y meningococcal vaccine is available as a conjugate (MenACWY [Menactra, Menveo]) or a polysaccharide (MPSV4 [Menomune]) vaccine.
  — Serogroup B meningococcal (MenB) vaccine is available as a 2-dose series of MenB-4C vaccine (Bexsero) administered at least 1 month apart or a 3-dose series of MenB-FHbp (Trumenba) vaccine administered at 0, 2, and 6 months; the two MenB vaccines are not interchangeable, i.e., the same MenB vaccine product must be used for all doses.
  — MenACWY vaccine is preferred for adults with serogroup A, C, W, and Y meningococcal vaccine indications who are aged ≤55 years, and for adults aged ≥56 years: 1) who were vaccinated previously with MenACWY vaccine and are recommended for revaccination or 2) for whom multiple doses of vaccine are anticipated; MPSV4 vaccine is preferred for adults aged ≥56 years who have not received MenACWY vaccine previously and who require a single dose only (e.g., persons at risk because of an outbreak).
  — Revaccination with MenACWY vaccine every 5 years is recommended for adults previously vaccinated with MenACWY or MPSV4 vaccine who remain at increased risk for infection (e.g., adults with anatomical for functional asplenia or persistent complement component deficiencies, or microbiologists who are routinely exposed to isolates of *Neisseria meningitidis*).
  — MenB vaccine is approved for use in persons aged 10 through 25 years; however, because there is no theoretical difference in safety for persons aged >25 years compared to those aged 10 through 25 years, MenB vaccine is recommended for routine use in persons aged ≥10 years who are at increased risk for serogroup B meningococcal disease.
  — There is no recommendation for MenB revaccination at this time.

Figure 6 Continued

47

- MenB vaccine may be administered concomitantly with MenACWY vaccine but at a different anatomic site, if feasible.
- HIV infection is not an indication for routine vaccination with MenACWY or MenB vaccine; if an HIV-infected person of any age is to be vaccinated, administer 2 doses of MenACWY vaccine at least 2 months apart.

- Adults with anatomical or functional asplenia or persistent complement component deficiencies: administer 2 doses of MenACWY vaccine at least 2 months apart and revaccinate every 5 years. Also administer a series of MenB vaccine.
- Microbiologists who are routinely exposed to isolates of *Neisseria meningitidis*: administer a single dose of MenACWY vaccine; revaccinate with MenACWY vaccine every 5 years if remain at increased risk for infection. Also administer a series of MenB vaccine.
- Persons at risk because of a meningococcal disease outbreak: if the outbreak is attributable to serogroup A, C, W, or Y, administer a single dose of MenACWY vaccine; if the outbreak is attributable to serogroup B, administer a series of MenB vaccine.
- Persons who travel to or live in countries in which meningococcal disease is hyperendemic or epidemic: administer a single dose of MenACWY vaccine and revaccinate with MenACWY vaccine every 5 years if the increased risk for infection remains (see footnote 1); MenB vaccine is not recommended because meningococcal disease in these countries is generally not caused by serogroup B.
- Military recruits: administer a single dose of MenACWY vaccine.
- First-year college students aged ≤21 years who live in residence halls: administer a single dose of MenACWY vaccine if they have not received a dose on or after their 16th birthday.
- Young adults aged 16 through 23 years (preferred age range is 16 through 18 years): may be vaccinated with a series of MenB vaccine to provide short-term protection against most strains of serogroup B meningococcal disease.

12. *Haemophilus influenza type b* (Hib) vaccination

- One dose of Hib vaccine should be administered to persons who have anatomical or functional asplenia or sickle cell disease or are undergoing elective splenectomy if they have not previously received Hib vaccine. Hib vaccination 14 or more days before splenectomy is suggested.
- Recipients of a hematopoietic stem cell transplant (HSCT) should be vaccinated with a 3-dose regimen 6–12 months after a successful transplant, regardless of vaccination history; at least 4 weeks should separate doses.
- Hib vaccine is not recommended for adults with HIV infection since their risk for Hib infection is low.

13. Immunocompromising conditions

- Inactivated vaccines (e.g., pneumococcal, meningococcal, and inactivated influenza vaccines) generally are acceptable and live vaccines generally should be avoided in persons with immune deficiencies or immunocompromising conditions. Information on specific conditions is available at www.cdc.goc/vaccines/hcp/acip-recs/index.html.

Figure 6 Continued

48

Table 6 SUMMARY OF VACCINES ROUTINELY RECOMMENDED FOR ADULTS

Vaccine	*Age Group*	*Dosing*
Td/Tdap (Tetanus, diphtheria, acellular pertussis)	19 years of age and older	1 dose of Tdap; Td booster every 10 years; pregnant women should receive a Tdap dose with each pregnancy
Influenza	All persons ≥ 6 months of age	1 dose annually
MMR (measles, mumps, rubella)	If born in 1957 or later (for those with no documentation of vaccination or clinical disease)	1–2 doses (0, 4–8 weeks)
Varicella	All persons ≥ 1 year of age lacking documentation of vaccination or clinical disease	2 doses (0, 4–8 weeks)
Herpes zoster (Shingles)	Persons ≥ 60 years of age with or without history of herpes zoster	1 dose
Pneumococcal polysaccharide (PPSV23)	Persons 2 years of age to 64 years in at-risk groups	1-2 doses (separated by 5 years)
	Persons ≥65 years	1 dose
Pneumococcccal conjugate (PCV13)	Persons ≥ 19 years of age with at risk conditions	1 dose
	Persons ≥65 years	1 dose

Table 6 CONTINUED

Vaccine	Age Group	Dosing
Hepatitis A	All children ≥ 1 year, all persons in at-risk groups or travelers	2 doses (0, 6–18 months)
Hepatitis B	All infants and children beginning at birth, persons in at-risk groups, travelers of any age	3 doses (0, 1, 6 months)
HPV	All persons 9 years to 26 years of age	3 doses (0, 1–2, 6 months)
Meningococcal quadrivalent conjugate	Adolescents	1–3 doses
	Persons in at-risk groups and travelers 9 months of age and older	1 or more doses

VACCINES AND PREGNANCY

Did you know that:

- During the 1917–1918 influenza pandemic in Chicago the mortality rate was 45% among hospitalized pregnant women with influenza.
- During the 2009 H1N1 influenza pandemic, pregnant women made up 1% of the US population but accounted for 5% of the deaths from the 2009 H1N1 influenza virus.

Over 91% of the deaths occurred during the second and third trimesters of pregnancy.

- If a woman contracts rubella during the first 10 weeks of pregnancy, the rate of transmission to the developing fetus is as high as 90%.
- The damage caused by a congenital rubella infection does not stop at birth; glaucoma, cataracts, retinal detachment, esophageal problems, autism, and thyroiditis may occur later in life.

Many infectious diseases are particularly threatening when they occur during pregnancy because of the serious complication rates that approach levels associated with those of high-risk populations. Many of these diseases are vaccine-preventable, some of which can directly affect a fetus at various stages of pregnancy.

The use of vaccines during pregnancy poses only theoretical risks to the developing fetus. There is no evidence that indicates that vaccines currently in use have detrimental effects on the fetus, however, the traditional approach to using vaccines during pregnancy has been that pregnant women should receive a vaccine only when the vaccine is unlikely to cause harm, risk of disease exposure is high, and the infection would pose a significant risk to the pregnant woman, fetus, or newborn infant. Two vaccines are now recommended for routine administration during pregnancy in the United States: inactivated influenza vaccines and Tdap. Diphtheria and tetanus toxoids (Td vaccine) may be indicated in some circumstances.

The American Congress of Obstetricians and Gynecologists (ACOG) and the Advisory Committee for Immunization Practice (ACIP) of the CDC have made strong recommendations for the use of vaccinations to improve the health of both mothers and infants. Table 7 details the vaccines that are routinely recommended, contraindicated, not recommended, or may be given in

Table 7 VACCINES IN PREGNANCY

Vaccines **routinely** given to pregnant women	Vaccines **contraindicated** during pregnancy	Vaccines **not** recommended during pregnancy	Vaccines **given** **in certain** **circumstances** during pregnancy
Td (late second or third trimester)	MMR	HPV	Hepatitis A
Tdap (late second or third trimester)	Live, attenuated, intranasal influenza (LAIV)		Hepatitis B
Inactivated injectable influenza (any trimester of pregnancy)	Varicella		Pneumococcal polysaccharide
	Herpes zoster		Meningococcal conjugate
			IPV

certain circumstances during pregnancy. Details of the individual VPDs are given in the specific vaccine book chapters.

Specific complications of VPDs in pregnant women and preventative vaccines and their use

Tdap (tetanus, diphtheria, acellular pertussis)
A tetanus containing vaccine can be given if indicated at any time during pregnancy, and the current recommendation is that it should be given as Tdap vaccine as noted below.

Pertussis (whooping cough) is particularly severe in infants especially during the first 3 months of life, when the vast majority of deaths from the disease occur. These infants are either too young to be immunized or have only received one dose of a pertussis containing vaccine and have little to no immunity against the disease. The disease is transmitted from any close contact, particularly family members (especially mothers, fathers, grandparents, and older siblings), care givers (nannies, babysitters, daycare providers), and visitors (aunts, uncles, friends). Infants begin their primary immunization schedule at 2 months of age when they receive their first dose of pertussis containing vaccine. The primary immunization schedule consists of 3 doses of a pertussis containing vaccine that is given at 2, 4, and 6 months of age. This leaves infants under 3 months of age at high risk for serious complications of the disease. To provide maximum protection to this young infant population, it is recommended that a pregnant woman receive a dose of Tdap vaccine during the late second or third trimester (between 27 and 36 weeks) of *each* pregnancy. If she was not immunized during the pregnancy and she has never received a prior dose of Tdap vaccine, she should receive the vaccine post-partum, as a one-time, single dose, as soon as possible after delivery and before leaving the hospital. She should be revaccinated with a dose of Tdap in all subsequent pregnancies.

It is also extremely important to vaccinate all susceptible family members and household contacts, as well as, other persons who have regular contact with the young infants including: daycare providers, nannies, family members, and visitors in order to prevent them from contracting pertussis. This protection cocoons the infant who is too young to be immunized and prevents the spread of the disease. Health-care workers that will have any direct contact with a patient should also be immunized.

Influenza

Pregnant women often have the highest rates of serious disease, complications, hospitalizations, and deaths from influenza. Pregnancy itself is considered an indication for influenza vaccination. The risk of hospitalization for heart and lung problems is more than 4 times higher in pregnant women compared to nonpregnant women and the risk increases exponentially as pregnancy progresses. The rate of complications, in otherwise healthy pregnant women, is similar to the high-risk nonpregnant patient. This risk is further increased in women with asthma who are pregnant. In the 2009 H1N1 epidemic, infected pregnant women were at very high risk for severe or fatal illness and were at significantly increased risk for fetal death, spontaneous abortion, and preterm delivery. Secondary bacterial pneumonia occurred much more commonly in this population and may be necrotizing, most often due to *Staphylococcus aureus* and *Streptococcus pneumoniae*. It is safe for a woman to receive all routine vaccines (both inactivated and live) immediately after giving birth; breastfeeding is not a precaution or contraindication to receiving a vaccine.

There are several different formulations and methods of administration for influenza vaccine that are available and are discussed in the appropriate chapter. All influenza vaccines contain the same three or four influenza strains that change on an annual basis. Only the inactivated injectable influenza vaccines are recommended to be given during pregnancy. ACOG strongly recommends that *all* women who will be pregnant during influenza season receive a dose of influenza vaccine. The vaccine may be given during *any* trimester of pregnancy.

Measles, mumps, and rubella

RUBEOLA (MEASLES)

This is usually a mild disease in children; however, in adults it can be associated with serious complications including pneumonia, encephalitis, and death. In pregnancy it can cause abortion, prematurity, and low birth weight. Immunity is important, since the disease is highly contagious, easily spread from an infected person, and can be imported from other countries where vaccination is not routinely recommended, as in the United States. Unvaccinated travelers returning from countries where vaccination is not widely done present significant risk to their community, particularly where there has been opposition to appropriate vaccination program.

MUMPS

Mumps are manifested as salivary gland swelling and tenderness; it has long been associated with orchitis and potential male infertility. However, oophoritis can occur in females also potentially reducing fertility. Early in pregnancy there is the possibility of spontaneous abortion. When the disease occurs late in pregnancy, there is the potential for preterm birth and low birth weight infants.

RUBELLA

Rubella was the first virus demonstrated as a teratogen, and there is a high risk of developing congenital rubella syndrome (CRS) if the infection occurs in the first trimester of pregnancy. The classic triad of CRS includes deafness, cataracts, and cardiac disease. Rubella infection in the mother may be asymptomatic or mildly symptomatic but can cross the placental barrier and cause defects in the developing fetus.

MMR (MEASLES, MUMPS, RUBELLA) VACCINE

This is a live, virus vaccine; administration is contraindicated during pregnancy. Susceptibility can be tested prior to the onset of pregnancy, particularly if the woman was born after 1957 and does not have proof of having had rubella disease or immunization. All women of childbearing age should be immunized. The patient should wait a month after vaccination to become pregnant. If the vaccine is given inadvertently in pregnancy, termination should *not* be recommended, as there is no evidence of effect on the fetus or clinical rubella in infants born to pregnant women who were inadvertently vaccinated. Postpartum, susceptible women should be immunized; there is no contraindication to vaccination with breast feeding.

Varicella
Because the effects of the varicella virus on the fetus are unknown, pregnant women should not be vaccinated. Nonpregnant women who are vaccinated should avoid becoming pregnant for 1 month after each vaccine dose. For persons without evidence of immunity, having a pregnant household member is not a contraindication for vaccination.

Hepatitis A
Hepatitis A causes fever, nausea, abdominal pain, and jaundice as a result of an acute, self-limiting liver infection. The virus is transmitted via the fecal-oral route after close contact with infected individuals, contaminated food or drinks. Although there is insufficient data to conclude that the vaccine is safe during pregnancy, there is no live virus component in the vaccine, so it is unlikely to cause harm to either the mother or fetus, and pregnant women should receive the vaccine if they are at high risk for infection.

Hepatitis B

Hepatitis B virus causes acute liver infection with inflammation, vomiting, and jaundice. It can be self-limited or result in chronic hepatitis associated with long-term sequelae including cirrhosis, liver failure, hepatocellular carcinoma, and death. The virus is transmitted by close contact with infected blood and body fluids.

Hepatitis B infection in pregnancy, both acute and chronic infection, is concerning because of the risk of vertical transmission to the fetus and newborn. All pregnant women should be screened prenatally for hepatitis B surface antigen (HBsAg) status as part of the standard prenatal labs that are obtained. Perinatally acquired hepatitis B is associated with the highest risk of developing chronic disease in the newborn. A three dose hepatitis B vaccine series should be started for pregnant women who have not been vaccinated previously and are at high risk of acquiring the disease, namely those with more than one sex partner during the previous 6 months, those evaluated or treated for an STD, those with a history of recent or current injection drug use, those having had an HBsAg-positive sex partner, or those living in a household with a contact infected with hepatitis B.

Pneumococcal disease

Streptococcus pneumoniae is associated with significant morbidity and mortality related to pneumonia, meningitis, and bacteremia. Risk factors for acquiring disease include: chronic heart disease, chronic lung disease (which includes asthma, diabetes, cigarette smoking, alcoholism, chronic liver disease, cerebral spinal fluid leaks, cochlear implants, congenital or acquired immunodeficiency), diseases requiring immunosuppressive therapy, sickle cell disease and other hemoglobinopathies, and functional or anatomic asplenia.

Observational studies of PPSV23 vaccine in pregnancy have shown no increases in spontaneous abortion, teratogenicity, or preterm labor, and a randomized trial of pregnant women receiving PPSV23 at 35 weeks' gestation showed no adverse effects. There is insufficient data to recommend routine administration of either PCV13 or PPSV23 during pregnancy. The CDC currently recommends PPSV23 for pregnant women who have a medical risk factor that places them at increased risk for invasive pneumococcal disease. The safety of pneumococcal polysaccharide vaccine during the first trimester of pregnancy has not been evaluated, although no adverse consequences have been reported among newborns whose mothers were inadvertently vaccinated early in pregnancy.

Meningococcal disease
Meningococcal vaccines—both quadrivalent polysaccharide and quadrivalent protein conjugate—are inactivated vaccines and have not been associated with adverse maternal or fetal outcomes, however, there is no data available on the safety of vaccination with the quadrivalent protein conjugate vaccine during pregnancy. Given the lack of safety data on quadrivalent meningococcal protein conjugate vaccine, the quadrivalent polysaccharide vaccine is recommended for use during pregnancy in selected high-risk situations.

Polio
Although no adverse effects of IPV have been documented among pregnant women or their fetuses, vaccination of pregnant women should be avoided on theoretical grounds. However, if a pregnant woman is at increased risk for infection and requires immediate protection against polio, IPV can be administered in accordance with the recommended schedules for adults.

Typhoid fever
No data have been reported on the use of any of the typhoid fever vaccines in pregnant women.

Japanese encephalitis
No controlled studies have assessed the safety, immunogenicity, or efficacy of Ixiaro in pregnant women. Preclinical studies of Ixiaro in pregnant rats did not show evidence of harm to the mother or fetus.

Yellow fever
Pregnancy is a precaution for yellow fever (YF) vaccine administration, compared with most other live vaccines, which are contraindicated in pregnancy. In areas where YF is endemic, or during outbreaks, the benefits of YF vaccination are likely to far outweigh the risk of potential transmission of vaccine virus to the fetus or infant. If travel is unavoidable, and the risks for YF virus exposure are felt to outweigh the vaccination risks, a pregnant woman should be vaccinated. If the risks for vaccination are felt to outweigh the risks for YF virus exposure, pregnant women should be issued a medical waiver to fulfill health regulations in the various countries. Although no specific data are available, a woman should wait 4 weeks after receiving YF vaccine before conceiving.

Rabies
Because of the potential consequences of inadequately managed rabies exposure, pregnancy is not considered a contraindication to post-exposure prophylaxis. Certain studies have indicated no increased incidence of abortion, premature births, or fetal abnormalities associated with rabies vaccination. If the risk of exposure to rabies is substantial, preexposure prophylaxis also might be

indicated during pregnancy. Rabies exposure or the diagnosis of rabies in the mother should not be regarded as justification for terminating the pregnancy.

Cholera vaccine
Live, attenuated oral cholera vaccine is not absorbed systemically following oral administration, and maternal use is not expected to result in fetal exposure to the drug. Breastfeeding is also not expected to result in exposure of the infant to the drug. The vaccine may be considered for use in pregnant women who may be traveling to and/or working in cholera-affected countries, as maternal cholera disease is associated with adverse pregnancy outcomes including fetal death. The vaccine strain may be shed in the stool of the vaccinated mother for at least 7 days, with a potential for transmission of the vaccine strain from the mother to infant during vaginal delivery.

Frequently asked questions

Is it safe to receive a flu shot during pregnancy and at any specific time in pregnancy?
Yes, flu vaccine can be given at any time in pregnancy. Influenza is particularly dangerous during pregnancy and can lead to serious complications and hospitalization. Severe complications can also occur in infants born to mothers with influenza.

If a patient is inadvertently given an MMR vaccine early in an unsuspected pregnancy should the pregnancy be terminated?
No. There have been no cases of congenital rubella syndrome associated with inadvertent MMR vaccination during pregnancy.

Should a pregnant woman who is traveling to a part of the world where yellow fever is endemic be vaccinated with yellow fever vaccine?

Pregnancy is a precaution for yellow fever (YF) vaccine administration. If travel is unavoidable, and the risks for YF virus exposure (endemic area or during outbreak) are felt to outweigh the vaccination risks, a pregnant woman should be vaccinated.

Should grandparents from out of town be vaccinated with Tdap before visiting their newborn grandchild?

Yes. If they have not been previously vaccinated, they should be vaccinated prior to the visit.

PART III

ROUTINE VACCINES FOR VACCINE-PREVENTABLE DISEASES

DIPHTHERIA

Did you know that:

- Abraham Lincoln had 4 sons, 2 died from vaccine preventable infectious diseases. Eddie, Lincoln's second son, died at the age of 2 from diphtheria. His third son, Willie, died at age 11 from typhoid fever.
- The only son of Dr. Abraham Jacobi, who is often referred to as the "father of American Pediatrics," died of diphtheria at age 8, a disease for his father was a recognized authority.
- Historical descriptions of diphtheria (throat membrane, neck swelling, and suffocation) first appeared in ancient Egyptian writings from the second millennium BC.
- In 1921 there were 206,000 cases of diphtheria in the United States, resulting in 15,520 deaths. 20% of children under 5 years of age died from diphtheria.

Diphtheria is caused by toxigenic strains of the gram-positive, non-spore forming, nonmotile, pleomorphic bacillus

Corynebacterium diphtheriae. The disease can have a variety of manifestations including: respiratory tract diphtheria, which presents as membranous nasopharyngitis or obstructive laryngotracheitis. Onset of the disease is abrupt, with sore throat, mild pharyngeal injection, and the development of a gray membrane on one or both tonsils with extension to the tonsillar pillars, uvula, soft palate, oropharynx, and nasopharynx with a bloody nasal discharge. Involvement of the larynx and bronchi presents with symptoms of hoarseness, dyspnea, respiratory stridor, a brassy cough, cyanosis, retractions, and respiratory distress. Diphtheria may also present as cutaneous, vaginal, conjunctival, or otic disease; and as mycotic aneurysms, septic arthritis, and osteomyelitis. Local infections are associated with low-grade fever, malaise, and the gradual onset of manifestations over 1 to 2 days. Extensive neck swelling with cervical lymphadenitis (bull neck) is a sign of severe disease that occurs more often in persons who are unimmunized or inadequately immunized. Diphtheria remains endemic in the former Soviet Union, Africa, Latin America, Haiti, Asia, the Middle East, and parts of Europe where childhood immunization coverage with diphtheria toxoid-containing vaccines is suboptimal.

Life-threatening complications of respiratory diphtheria include upper airway obstruction caused by extensive membrane formation; myocarditis (detected in up to two-thirds of patients), which is often associated with varying degrees of heart block and myocardial dysfunction; cranial and peripheral neuropathies; and palatal palsy associated with pharyngeal diphtheria characterized by nasal speech.

Transmission

Humans are the sole reservoir of *C. diphtheriae*. Organisms are spread by intimate contact with airborne respiratory tract droplets from persons with active infection or carriers and by contact with exudates from infected skin lesions. People who travel to areas where diphtheria is endemic or people who come into contact with infected travelers from such areas are at increased risk of being infected with the organism.

Incubation period

2 to 7 days

Prevention

Postexposure

a. Persons who have diphtheria disease and are in the convalescent stage of their disease should receive a dose of a diphtheria toxoid-containing vaccine because clinical infection does not always induce adequate levels of antitoxin.

b. Close contacts of persons with diphtheria disease, regardless of their immunization status, should receive antibiotic prophylaxis with erythromycin or penicillin, *and* should receive a dose of a diphtheria toxoid-containing vaccine.

Preexposure

a. Diphtheria toxoid-containing vaccines—type of vaccine varies by age

    i. For infants and children from 6 weeks up to 7 years of age—5 intramuscular doses of DTaP vaccines are recommended, beginning at 6 to 8 weeks of age. Recommended doses are given at 2 months, 4 months, 6 months, 12 to 18 months and 4 to 6 years of age.

ii. For persons over 7 years of age—An intramuscular dose of Td vaccine should be administered if immunization against diphtheria or tetanus is indicated. A dose of Tdap vaccine (contains acellular pertussis) may also be given if a previous dose has not been received. Booster doses of Td are recommended every 10 years. Currently only a single dose of Tdap is recommended, however, discussions are underway regarding recommendation for booster doses.

Duration of immunity

approximately 10 years

Contraindications and precautions to diphtheria containing vaccines

Contraindications

Severe immediate allergic reaction (e.g., anaphylaxis) to a prior dose of tetanus and diphtheria toxoid-containing vaccines (e.g., DTaP, Tdap, Td) is a contraindication to further doses.

Precautions

1. Moderate or severe acute illness with or without fever
2. Guillain-Barré syndrome (GBS) within 6 weeks after a previous dose of tetanus-toxoid-containing vaccine
3. History of Arthus-type hypersensitivity reactions after a previous dose of tetanus or diphtheria toxoid-containing vaccine; defer vaccination until at least 10 years have elapsed since the last tetanus-toxoid-containing vaccine

Frequently asked questions

Diphtheria is rare in the United States, are there countries where diphtheria is still prevalent?

Yes, there are countries where diphtheria is still prevalent and poses a risk. These include countries in Asia (the Philippines, Nepal, Indonesia, Bangladesh, Vietnam), Africa, the Middle East (Pakistan, India, Afghanistan), the countries of the former Soviet Union (Russia, Ukraine, the Baltic States, and Georgia), South America, the South Pacific, Eastern Europe, Haiti, and the Dominican Republic. Persons traveling to these countries should ensure that they are up to date with their diphtheria toxoid vaccination status.

Who is at risk of acquiring diphtheria?

Persons, especially children who are not immunized or who did not receive adequate immunization are at the highest risk. Diphtheria is most common in areas where people live in crowded conditions with poor sanitation.

If a person is infected with diphtheria, how long are they contagious and able to spread disease to others?

Untreated people who are infected with the diphtheria organism can be contagious for up to two weeks but rarely more than four weeks. If treated with appropriate antibiotics, the contagious period can be limited to less than four days.

What are the potential consequences of not being treated for diphtheria?

If diphtheria goes untreated, serious complications such as paralysis, encephalitis, cerebral infarction, heart failure, and renal failure may occur. Death occurs in approximately 5% to 10% of all cases.

Does past infection with diphtheria make a person immune to the disease?
Unfortunately, a person who recovers from diphtheria does not reliably develop lasting immunity to the disease.

TETANUS

Did you know that:

- John Augustus Roebling, the architect of the Brooklyn Bridge, died from tetanus after his leg was crushed by a ferryboat while working on the bridge.
- John Thoreau, brother of famous American writer and Transcendentalist Henry David Thoreau, died from tetanus after cutting himself shaving.
- Tetanus is called "lockjaw" because one of the first symptoms of the disease is severe muscle spasms of the jaw muscles preventing opening of the mouth.

Tetanus (lockjaw) occurs worldwide and is more common in warmer climates and during warmer months. It is caused by neurotoxin produced by the anaerobic, spore forming, gram positive bacterium *Clostridium tetani*, which is a normal inhabitant of soil, animal, and human intestines, and is ubiquitous in the environment. The organism multiplies in wounds and elaborates toxins in the presence of anaerobic conditions. Contaminated wounds, especially wounds with devitalized tissue and deep-puncture trauma, are at greatest risk (including frostbite). Neonatal tetanus is common in many developing countries where pregnant women are not immunized appropriately against tetanus and nonsterile umbilical cord-care practices are followed.

Tetanus has 4 clinical forms:

1. Generalized tetanus (lockjaw) is a neurologic disease manifesting as severe muscle spasms including trismus (jaw muscle spasms or lockjaw), *risus sardonicus* (facial muscle spasms resulting in a sardonic grin), and opisthotonus (severe spasm and hyperextension of the neck and spine). Onset is gradual, occurring over 1 to 7 days, and symptoms rapidly progress to severe generalized muscle spasms, which are made worse by any external stimuli. Severe spasms persist for 1 or more weeks and subside over several weeks in persons who survive. Other symptoms include fever, diaphoresis, tachycardia, and elevated blood pressure associated with sympathetic overactivity.

2. Local tetanus manifests as local muscle spasms in areas contiguous to a contaminated wound that very often progresses to generalized tetanus.

3. Neonatal tetanus is a form of generalized tetanus occurring in newborn infants who lack protective passive immunity because their mothers are not immunized. Neonates present with generalized weakness and failure to nurse followed by apnea, rigidity, and spasms. Mortality rate exceeds 90%, and developmental delays are common among survivors.

4. Cephalic tetanus is a dysfunction of cranial nerves associated with infected wounds on the head and neck. Cephalic tetanus can progress to generalized tetanus.

Transmission

Contamination of wounds. The vegetative form of *C. tetani* produces a potent plasmid-encoded exotoxin (tetanospasmin), which binds to gangliosides at the myoneuronal junction of skeletal muscle and on neuronal membranes in the spinal cord, blocking inhibitory impulses to motor neurons.

Incubation period

The incubation period is 3 to 21 days, with the majority of cases occurring within 8 days. Shorter incubation periods are associated with more heavily contaminated wounds, more severe disease, and a worse prognosis. For neonatal tetanus, symptoms appear on average 7 days after birth (range 4 to 14 days).

Prevention

Postexposure

a. Tetanus toxoid-containing vaccine with or without human tetanus immunoglobulin (TIG) in the management of wounds depends on the type of wound and the immunization history with tetanus toxoid (Table 8). DTaP is used for children younger than 7 years of age. Tdap is preferred over Td for underimmunized persons over 7 years of age who have not received a prior dose of Tdap.

When an infant is born outside the hospital and the umbilical cord is likely contaminated (e.g., cut with nonsterile equipment), the maternal history of tetanus immunization should be confirmed. If the mother's tetanus immunization status is unknown and she

Table 8 MANAGEMENT OF WOUNDS DEPENDING ON WOUND TYPE AND TETANUS TOXOID IMMUNIZATION HISTORY

Number of Tetanus Toxoid Doses	Clean, Minor Wounds		All Other Wounds	
	DTaP/Tdap/Td	TIG	DTaP/Tdap/Td	TIG
≤ 3 or unknown	Yes	No	Yes	Yes
3 or more	**No** if <10 years since last tetanus containing vaccine	No	**No** if <5 years since last tetanus containing vaccine	No
	Yes if >10 years since last tetanus containing vaccine	No	**Yes** if ≥5 years since last tetanus containing vaccine	No

is unlikely to have been immunized, TIG should be administered to the neonate unless the maternal tetanus serostatus can be confirmed quickly.

For infants younger than 6 months of age who have not received a full 3-dose primary series of tetanus-toxoid-containing vaccine, decisions on the need for TIG with wound care should be based on the mother's tetanus toxoid immunization history at the time of delivery.

Preexposure

a. Active immunization with tetanus toxoid containing vaccine is recommended for persons of all ages. Tetanus immunization is administered with diphtheria toxoid containing vaccines (e.g., Td) or with diphtheria toxoid and acellular pertussis containing vaccines (e.g., DTaP,

Tdap)—type of vaccine varies by age. Vaccines are administered intramuscularly.

i. For infants and children from 6 weeks up to 7 years of age—5 intramuscular doses of DTaP vaccines are recommended, beginning at 6 to 8 weeks of age. Recommended doses are given at 2 months, 4 months, 6 months, 12 to 18 months and 4 to 6 years of age.

ii. For persons ≥ 7 years of age—an intramuscular dose of Td vaccine is given if immunization against diphtheria or tetanus is needed. A dose of Tdap vaccine (contains acellular pertussis) may also be given if a previous dose has not been received. Booster doses of Td are recommended every 10 years. Currently only a single dose of Tdap is recommended, however, discussions are underway regarding an appropriate interval for booster doses.

Duration of immunity

approximately 10 years

Contraindications and Precautions

Contraindications

Severe immediate allergic reaction (e.g., anaphylaxis) to a prior dose of tetanus and diphtheria toxoid-containing vaccines (e.g. DTaP, Tdap, Td) is a contraindication to further doses.

Precautions

1. Moderate or severe acute illness with or without fever
2. Guillain-Barré syndrome (GBS) within 6 weeks after a previous dose of tetanus-toxoid containing vaccine
3. History of Arthus-type hypersensitivity reactions after a previous dose of tetanus or diphtheria toxoid-containing vaccine; defer vaccination until at least 10 years have elapsed since the last tetanus-toxoid containing vaccine.

Frequently asked questions

If a person sustains a puncture wound or laceration that is tetanus prone (e.g., wounds contaminated with soil or fecal material), does the person need to receive tetanus wound management the day that the injury occurred or can this wait for 48 to 72 hours?

Puncture wounds should be attended to as soon as possible. The decision to delay a booster dose of tetanus-toxoid-containing vaccine following an injury should be based on the type of injury and likelihood that the person is susceptible to tetanus. The more likely the person is to be susceptible (e.g., unvaccinated or incompletely vaccinated against tetanus), the more quickly the tetanus prophylaxis (TIG and Tdap/Td) should be administered.

When should tetanus immue globulin (TIG) be administered as part of wound management?

TIG is recommended for any wound other than a clean minor wound if the person's vaccination history is either unknown, or if they have had less than a complete series of 3 doses of Td vaccine. TIG should be given as soon as possible after the injury.

How long after a wound occurs is tetanus immune globulin (TIG) no longer recommended?

For a person who has been vaccinated but is not up to date, there is little benefit in giving TIG more than a week after the injury. For a person who is completely vaccinated, this interval can be increased to up to day 21 post-injury period.

If an adult patient states that he/she had tetanus infection as a child but does not know if he/she have ever received any tetanus-containing vaccines, should this patient be immunized with a tetanus containing vaccine as part of routine health maintenance?

A history of tetanus disease is not a reason to avoid using tetanus-containing vaccines. Tetanus disease does not produce immunity because only a very small amount of toxin is needed to produce disease. If the patient has no other contraindications, they should receive a tetanus-containing vaccine now. If they have no documentation of prior tetanus vaccination, they should complete a 3-dose series with Tdap, followed by a dose of Td 4 to 8 weeks later, and a dose of Td 6-12 months after the last Td dose.

Should an adult patient who previously received a Tdap vaccine, receive another Tdap vaccine after a bone marrow transplant?

Yes. A dose of Tdap vaccine 6 months after a bone marrow transplant is appropriate.

Can Tdap and RhoGam (anti-Rho[D]) immunoglobulin be given at the same prenatal visit?

Yes. Tdap is an inactivated vaccine and may be given at the same prenatal visit with RhoGam.

PERTUSSIS

Did you know that:

- George Washington Carver (American botanist and inventor), Dolly Madison (wife of US President James Madison), and Shah Mohammed Reza Pahlavi (the Shah of Iran) all suffered from bouts of pertussis.
- Pertussis is also known as "whooping cough" because of the "whooping" sound that is made when gasping for air after a fit of coughing.
- Coughing fits due to pertussis infection can last for up to 10 weeks or more; this disease has been called the "cough of 100 days."

Pertussis (whooping cough) is caused by the Gram negative organism *Bordetella pertussis*. Humans are the only known hosts of the organism. It continues to be a major public health problem in all age groups and is the cause of major epidemics worldwide. Cases occur year round. The incidence of disease in the adolescent and adult populations has significantly increased over the last several decades primarily due to waning of both vaccine and naturally induced immunity and increased disease awareness. Neither natural infection nor immunization provides lifelong immunity. Older children, adolescents, and adults serve as the major reservoirs of pertussis disease in the community. Young infants, especially those under 3 months of age, are at the greatest risk for morbidity and mortality from disease. Since 1990, 93% to 100% of pertussis deaths in the United States have occurred in this very young infant population. The CDC, AAP, IOM, AAFP, and ACOG all strongly support immunization of pregnant women and a "cocoon strategy" to protect these young infants. This strategy

Table 9 CLINICAL SIGNS AND SYMPTOMS OF PERTUSSIS IN ADOLESCENTS AND ADULTS (BASED ON A COMPILATION OF 8 DIFFERENT STUDIES)

	Age Group	
Clinical Characteristics	Adolescents (%) (10 to 19 years)	Adults (%) (≥20 years)
Paroxysms of cough	82.5 (82–83)	87 (33–100)
Inspiratory whoop	50 (30–67)	74 (7–82)
Apnea	46 (19–86)	85 (29–87)
Cyanosis	6–15	9–12
Posttussive emesis	56 (45–71)	50 (17–70)
Hospitalization	1.4–7.5	3.5–5.7

focuses on the targeted immunization of older children, adolescents, and adults who either live in the household or who are close contacts of these young infants to prevent these individuals from getting pertussis disease and giving it to the young infants. This should include all adolescents and adults including persons over 65 years of age, grandparents, relatives, friends, nannies, babysitters, daycare providers, and housekeepers.

Pertussis disease consists of 3 stages and severity of disease ranges from very mild, atypical disease to severe classic pertussis (Table 9):

Stage 1: Catarrhal stage—symptoms are mild and include rhinorrhea with no pharyngitis, mild conjunctival injection, low-grade fever or no fever and mild cough. This stage lasts for 2 weeks.

Stage 2: Paroxysmal stage—symptoms include paroxysms of cough, posttussive emesis, inspiratory whooping, apnea, and cyanosis. Symptoms may be milder in individuals who have received immunization in the past and in the adolescent and adult populations. This stage lasts for 6 weeks.

Stage 3: Convalescent stage—coughing paroxysms and other symptoms become less frequent and intense. This stage lasts for 4-6 weeks.

Persons with pertussis may be ill for 3 to 4 months from onset of cough. Any intercurrent viral illness will exacerbate cough illness. Treatment with antibiotic therapy is effective in preventing transmission of the organism but does not have an impact on the duration of the cough. The illness has a significant negative impact on the quality of life of adolescent and adult patients with pertussis. The vast majority are unable to sleep, go to work, attend school, eat or drink normally during their illness.

Pertussis should be included in the differential diagnosis for all adolescents and adults presenting for evaluation of a persistent cough illness lasting 2 weeks or more.

Infants, especially those under 3 months of age, who are unimmunized or who have received only the first of their primary immunizations, are at the greatest risk for complications, hospitalizations, and death due to pertussis disease. Apnea alone or apnea associated with very mild cough may be the only presenting symptom of pertussis in this age group. Complications seen among infants include: pneumonia (22%), seizures (2%), encephalopathy (<0.5%), pulmonary hypertension, hernia, subdural bleeding, conjunctival bleeding and death.

Complications in children, adolescents, and adults

These complications include pneumonia (1.9% in patients <30 years of age, 5% to 9% in older patients), seizures (0.3%), encephalopathy (0.1%), urinary incontinence (4% of adults, 35% of women >50 years), pneumothorax, inguinal hernia, aspiration pneumonia, fractured ribs, hearing loss, syncope, subconjunctival hemorrhages, carotid artery dissection, and intracranial bleeding. Incidence of complications increases with age.

Table 10 ANTIBIOTIC TREATMENT AND CHEMOPROPHYLAXIS OF PERTUSSIS

Antibiotic	Dosage	Comments
Erythromycin estolate or erythromycin ethylsuccinate	40–50 mg/kg/day (max 2 g/day) PO divided q 6–8 hours X 14 days	Contraindicated in infants <6 weeks of age due to increased risk for pyloric stenosis
Azithromycin	10 mg/kg/day X 5 days (infants <6 mos); 10 mg/kg on day 1 (max 500 mg/day) then 5 mg/kg per day on days 2–5 (max 250 mg/day)	DRUG OF CHOICE FOR ALL AGE GROUPS
Clarithromycin	15–20 mg/kg/day (max 1 gram/day) q 8–12 hours X 7–10 days	___
Trimethoprim-sulfamethoxazole (TMP/SMX)	8 mg TMP/40 mg SMX per kg/day (max 320 mg TMP/1600 mg SMX/day) in 2 divided doses X 14 days	Drug of choice for patients who cannot tolerate the macrolide antibiotics or who are allergic to the macrolide antibiotics

Persons who should receive chemoprophylaxis include:

- All household contacts **regardless of age and immunization status**
- Other close contacts regardless of age and immunization status defined by the CDC as:
  - Anyone who has had face-to-face contact or shared a confined space for a prolonged period of time (>1 hour) with an infected individual
  - Persons who have direct contact with respiratory, oral, or nasal secretions from a symptomatic patient (e.g., cough, sneeze, sharing food and eating utensils, mouth-to-mouth resuscitation, or performing a medical examination of the mouth, nose, and throat)

Transmission

Close contact with cases via aerosolized respiratory droplets. Persons are infectious beginning with the first day of cough and if untreated can continue to transmit the organism for up to 3 weeks after onset of illness.

Prevention

Postexposure

a. Antibiotic chemoprophylaxis for all household and close contacts as above in addition to pertussis containing vaccines.

b. Pertussis containing vaccines are recommended for all underimmunized or incompletely immunized household and close contacts. Pertussis immunization is administered with diphtheria and tetanus-toxoid- containing vaccines (e.g., DTaP, Tdap)—type of vaccine varies by age.

Vaccines are administered intramuscularly. DTaP is used for children younger than 7 years of age. Tdap is used for underimmunized persons over 7 years of age who have not received a prior dose of Tdap.

Preexposure

Pertussis containing vaccines

i. For infants and children from 6 weeks up to 7 years of age—5 intramuscular doses of DTaP vaccines are recommended, beginning at 6 to 8 weeks of age. Recommended doses are given at 2 months, 4 months, 6 months, 12–18 months and 4 to 6 years of age.

ii. For persons over 7 years of age—an intramuscular dose of Tdap vaccine is given if immunization against pertussis is needed and if a previous dose has not been received. Currently only a single dose of Tdap is recommended, except in the case of pregnant women, however, discussions are underway regarding interval for boosting.

iii. It is recommended that pregnant women receive a dose of Tdap vaccine after 20 weeks' gestation (during the late second or third trimesters of pregnancy) for each pregnancy, regardless of prior immunization status or time interval since previous Tdap dose.

iv. If a woman is unable to receive a dose of Tdap during pregnancy, postpartum administration of a dose of Tdap is a viable option for those women who have not received a previous Tdap dose. The dose should be given as soon as possible after delivery but before hospital discharge.

    v. Tdap vaccine is recommended for all adolescents starting at 11 to 12 years of age and all adults **regardless** of the interval from the last dose of Td vaccine.

   vi. Tdap vaccine is strongly recommended for all health-care workers that have any direct patient contact either in a hospital or clinic setting **regardless** of the interval from the last dose of Td vaccine.

Duration of immunity

The duration is 3 to 5 years after last dose of pertussis containing vaccine. Immunity is at best 10 years after natural infection.

Contraindications and precautions

Contraindications

1. Encephalopathy (e.g., coma, decreased level of consciousness, prolonged seizures) not attributable to another identifiable cause within 7 days of administration of a previous dose of DTP or DTaP (for DTaP); or a previous dose of DTP, DTaP, or Tdap (Tdap).
2. Severe immediate allergic reaction (e.g., anaphylaxis) to a prior dose of vaccine or to a vaccine component

Precautions

1. Moderate or severe acute illness with or without fever
2. Guillain-Barré syndrome (GBS) within 6 weeks after a previous dose of tetanus-toxoid-containing vaccine
3. Progressive or unstable neurologic disorder (including infantile spasms for DTaP), uncontrolled seizures, or progressive encephalopathy until a treatment regimen has been established and the condition has stabilized.

4. For DTaP only:

    a. Temperature of 105°F or higher (40.5°C or higher) within 48 hours after vaccination with a previous dose of DTP/DTaP

    b. Collapse or shock-like state (i.e., hypotonic hyporesponsive episode) within 48 hours after receiving a previous dose of DTP/DTaP

    c. Seizure within 3 days after receiving a previous dose of DTP/DTaP

    d. Persistent, inconsolable crying lasting 3 or more hours within 48 hours after receiving a previous dose of DTP/DTaP

Frequently asked questions

If a person (infant, child, or adult) has had a documented case of pertussis, can they get the disease again?
Reinfection is uncommon but it does occur. Symptoms with reinfection may present as only a persistent cough with little else.

If a person (infant, child, adolescent, or adult) has had pertussis disease, should they still be vaccinated with a pertussis-containing vaccine?
Yes. All persons who have a history of pertussis disease generally should receive pertussis-containing vaccines (DTaP or Tdap) according to the routine schedule. This is recommended because the amount and duration of protection induced by pertussis disease is unknown and because the diagnosis of pertussis can be difficult to confirm.

Which HCWs should be vaccinated against pertussis with tetanus-diphtheria-acellular pertussis (Tdap) vaccine?
The CDC recommends that all HCWs, regardless of age, should receive a dose of Tdap as soon as feasible if they have not previously received Tdap and regardless of the time since their last Td vaccine.

If a health-care worker (HCW) has been vaccinated with tetanus-diphtheria-acellular pertussis (Tdap) vaccine and is then has a significant exposure to someone with pertussis, does the vaccinated HCW need to be treated with prophylactic antibiotics or are they considered immune to the disease?
All HCWs who have a significant exposure to pertussis disease should receive antibiotic prophylaxis regardless of their immunization status. Effectiveness of Tdap in preventing pertussis in the health-care setting is currently unknown. Until studies can be performed that define the optimal management of exposed vaccinated HCWs, the CDC's post-exposure prophylaxis protocol for pertussis exposure should be followed.

How many doses of pediatric diphtheria-tetanus-acellular pertussis (DTaP) vaccine does an infant need before they are protected from pertussis?
Vaccine efficacy following 3 doses of pediatric DTaP vaccine is 80% to 85%. Information regarding efficacy after 1 or 2 doses is limited, but efficacy is most likely lower. In order to protect the infant against pertussis prior to them receiving their 3-dose primary DTaP vaccine series, it is important that all people who live in the household with the infant and all those

who provide care to them (e.g., babysitters, nannies, au pairs, and daycare providers) be protected against pertussis. It is recommended that these individuals receive a dose of adolescent/adult tetanus-diphtheria-acellular pertussis vaccine (Tdap) if they have not already done so.

What should be done in the situation where a 4-month-old infant inadvertently received a dose of adolescent/adult Tdap instead of pediatric DTaP?

If Tdap is inadvertently administered to a child under 7 years of age, it should *not* be counted as valid for the first, second, or third dose of DTaP (primary vaccine series). The dose should be repeated with a dose of DTaP and the routine vaccination schedule should be followed. If the dose of Tdap was administered for the fourth or fifth booster dose, the Tdap dose can be counted as valid.

What should be done in the situation where a 10-year-old child inadvertently received a dose of DTaP instead of Tdap?

DTaP given to patients age 7 years or older can be counted as valid for the Tdap dose.

What should be done in the situation where a 12-year-old patient received only 2 doses of DTP (whole cell pertussis vaccine) at 2 months and 4 months of age after developing persistent crying and a temperature of 105°F following the second dose of DTP vaccine. Is it safe to give this patient a dose of Tdap vaccine?

Yes, it is safe to give a dose of Tdap vaccine. Many of the precautions to DTP and DTaP (e.g., temperature of 105°F or higher, persistent crying lasting 3 hours of longer, seizure with or without fever, and hyporesponsive or shock-like state) do not apply to the Tdap vaccine.

A 2-month old received her first dose of DTaP vaccine and then developed inconsolable crying for greater than 3 hours. Should the infant receive additional doses of DTaP or should they be given DT vaccine?

Persistent crying following DTaP has been observed much less frequently than it was following the use of DTP (whole cell pertussis) vaccine. When it occurs following DTaP, it is considered a precaution. If the benefit of the pertussis vaccine exceeds the risk of persistent crying (which in itself is benign), one can administer additional doses of DTaP. Many providers choose to administer pertussis-containing vaccine if this is the only precaution the infant has experienced. The health-care provider and the parent will need to make this judgement.

Is there an upper age limit for Tdap administration?

There is *no* upper age limit for Tdap vaccination. A single dose of Tdap is recommended for all adults regardless of age.

Which adults should be vaccinated with a Tdap vaccine?

The CDC recommends that *all* adults age 19 years and older receive a dose of Tdap vaccine regardless of the interval since the last tetanus or diphtheria-toxoid containing vaccine (e.g., Td).

What should be done in the situation where a patient remembers receiving a "tetanus booster" several years ago at a convenient care clinic but no vaccination record is

available and the patient does not remember if he received Td or Tdap. The patient's wife is 37 weeks pregnant. Can the patient receive a dose of Tdap vaccine as a way to protect their soon to be born child against pertussis?

Yes. If vaccination is indicated and there is a lack of vaccine documentation, a dose of Tdap can be given to the patient.

If a pregnant woman got a dose of Td during pregnancy, how soon can she get her dose of Tdap?

She should have been given Tdap rather than Td; however, she can receive her Tdap *at any interval* since the Td dose was given, preferably between 27 and 36 weeks gestation.

If a woman received a dose of Tdap early in her pregnancy (e.g., in her first trimester), should she get another dose in the third trimester?

No, it is not recommended to give another dose of Tdap. The optimal timing for Tdap administration in pregnancy is between 27 and 36 weeks' gestation because of the favorable transplacental antibody kinetics. Tdap may be administered at any time during pregnancy, but vaccination during the third trimester would provide the highest concentration of maternal antibodies to be transferred.

Should fathers and other family members receive a Tdap booster each time there is a pregnancy in the family to boost the cocoon effect to protect the newborn from pertussis?

At this time the CDC does not recommend additional doses of Tdap vaccine for fathers, other family members or caregivers. The recommendation for a dose of Tdap with each pregnancy only applies to the pregnant woman.

Can Tdap vaccine be given to breastfeeding mothers?

Yes. Women who have never received Tdap and who did not receive it during pregnancy should receive it immediately post-partum or as soon as feasibly possible. Breastfeeding does not decrease the immune response to routine childhood vaccine.

My practice is seeing a number of patients who are refugees or who have immigrated from other countries. What vaccine schedule should be used to vaccinate children, adolescents, or adults who have never received the primary series of tetanus-toxoid-containing vaccines?

Children 7 years of age and older, adolescents and adults who have never received tetanus-containing vaccines, or whose vaccination history is unknown, should receive a 3-dose vaccine series. The CDC recommends Tdap at 0, and Td at 4 weeks and at least 6 months. Tdap can be substituted for only one of the 3 Td doses in the series, preferably the first. The amount of protection provided by a single dose of Tdap in a person who has not previously received pertussis vaccine is not known. Following the primary series, booster doses of Td should be given every 10 years.

If a child has already received 5 appropriately spaced doses of DTaP (6-month intervals between doses #3 and #4 and doses #4 and #5) by their fourth birthday, should a booster dose be given after the fourth birthday?

As a rule, a child should receive no more than 4 doses of DTaP before 4 years of age. The CDC recommends that a dose of DTaP be given at 4 to 6 years of age. Many states have school immunization laws which require that at least one dose of DTP/DTaP be given on or after the fourth birthday. This dose is important to boost immunity to pertussis.

INFLUENZA

Did you know that:

- The word "influenza" comes from the Italian *influentia* because it was believed that the influence of the planets, moon, and stars caused the flu—for only such universal influence could explain such sudden and widespread illness.
- Martin van Buren, the eighth president of the United States; Benjamin Harrison, the twenty-third president of the United States; Juan Peron, the former president of Argentina; Shoghi Effendi, the Guardian and appointed head of the Baha'i faith; and Sir William Osler, physician, educator, and medical philosopher all died from severe influenza infections.
- The Spanish influenza pandemic of 1918 killed between 20 to 40 million people, which is more than the number that were killed during World War I. More people died in one year from this pandemic than in 4 years of the Black Death Bubonic Plague from 1347 to 1351. The death rate for 15 to 34-year-olds of influenza and pneumonia were 20 times higher in 1918 than in previous years. People were struck with illness on the street and died rapid deaths—"people on their way to work suddenly developing the flu and dying within hours."

Influenza causes annual epidemics during the winter months with up to 20% of the US population becoming ill with influenza A or B viruses. Children are the most likely to acquire and transmit infection given that they are able to shed virus at very high titers and for prolonged periods of time (≥10 days). Up to 40% of healthy children become ill with influenza each year. However, the populations with the highest rates of serious disease, complications and deaths are persons ≥65 years of age, children <2 years of age, pregnant women, and persons of any age with underlying medical conditions. Each year, complications from influenza are responsible for >200,000 hospitalizations and an average of 36,000 deaths, with greater than 50% of the hospitalizations and 90% of the deaths occurring in persons ≥65 years of age. On a societal level, influenza is an extraordinarily expensive disease with an average of $10 billion dollars being spent each year on health care and work-loss costs.

The clinical presentation of influenza differs by age. The typical symptoms of the sudden onset of fever accompanied by chills or rigors, headache, malaise, diffuse myalgia, non-productive cough, sore throat, nasal congestion, and rhinorrhea are seen most commonly in the adolescent and adult populations. Children more commonly have fever, non-productive cough, rhinitis, nasal congestion, nausea, vomiting, abdominal pain and diarrhea. Symptoms in the elderly population are very nonspecific with cough and malaise being the most common. Symptoms in all age groups usually resolve after 3 to 7 days; however, cough and malaise may persist for >2 weeks.

Persons at increased risk for influenza complications

- Children 6 to 59 months of age
- Adults ≥ 50 years of age (especially persons ≥65 years of age)
- Pregnant women
- Adults and children with chronic pulmonary, renal, cardiovascular, hepatic, neurologic, hematologic, or metabolic disorders
- Immunosuppressed patients (immunosuppressive medications, HIV infection)

- Residents in long-term care facilities (of any age)
- Health-care personnel
- Morbidly obese people, BMI ≥40 kg/m²
- Household contacts and caregivers of children <5 years (especially <6 months of age) and adults ≥50 years
- Children and adolescents (6 months to 18 years) receiving long-term aspirin therapy

  Immunization rates for all these at risk populations are well below the levels recommended by the Healthy People 2020 Goals.

Complications of influenza in the adult population

These complications include primary influenza pneumonia and/ or secondary bacterial pneumonia, which may be necrotizing and is most often due to *Staphylococcus aureus* and *Streptococcus pneumoniae*; pneumonia may be especially severe in pregnant women; exacerbation of underlying pulmonary or cardiac disease; encephalitis; myositis; myocarditis; pericarditis; transverse myelitis; Guillain-Barré syndrome. Complications of influenza in the pediatric population include: acute otitis media; bronchiolitis; laryngotracheobronchitis; bacterial pneumonia, which may be necrotizing and is most often due to *Staphylococcus aureus* and *Streptococcus pneumoniae*; encephalitis and encephalopathy, which may be necrotizing; dehydration with severe hypotension; respiratory failure; myositis; transverse myelitis.

Influenza can be particularly severe in pregnant women. The risk of hospitalization for heart and lung problems is more than 4X higher in pregnant women compared to non-pregnant women and the risk increases exponentially as pregnancy progresses. This risk is further increased in women with asthma who are pregnant. For example, pregnant women infected with the 2009

H1N1 influenza virus were at very high risk for severe or fatal illness and were at significantly increased risk for fetal death, spontaneous abortions, and preterm delivery. In 2009 pregnant women represented 1% of the US population but accounted for 5% of the US deaths from H1N1 disease. Over 91% of the deaths occurred in women in their second and third trimesters of pregnancy.

Transmission

Person to person by respiratory droplets or by direct contact with articles contaminated with nasopharyngeal secretions via coughing and sneezing

Incubation period

Incubation period is 1 to 4 days (average 2 days). Adults are infectious from the day before symptoms begin through 5 days after illness onset. Children are infectious for several days before onset of symptoms through ≥10 days after illness onset.

Prevention

Post-exposure
   a. Influenza vaccine is the primary means of protecting persons against influenza disease and its complications, and can be administered at any time during influenza season, even when the virus is circulating in the community. Vaccines may be trivalent or quadrivalent. The trivalent vaccines contain two influenza A strains and one influenza B strain—there are several different formulations of the vaccine and method of administration that are available.

Quadrivalent influenza vaccine (containing two influenza A strains and two influenza B strains) became available beginning in the 2013–2014 influenza season. Injectable and intranasal formations are available for this vaccine.

b. Chemoprophylaxis with influenza antiviral drugs is an adjunctive measure, *not* a substitute, for immunization. It may be used in certain situations in order to control and prevent influenza disease. Situations in which chemoprophylaxis may be considered include:

- Protection of unimmunized high-risk children or adults or children or adults who were immunized less than 2 weeks before influenza circulation in the community
- Protection of children and adults at increased risk of severe infection or complications, such as high-risk populations for whom the vaccine is contraindicated
- Protection of unimmunized close contacts of persons at high risk
- Protection of immunocompromised persons who may not respond to vaccine
- Control of influenza outbreaks in a closed setting, such as an institution with unimmunized high-risk persons
- Protection of immunized high-risk persons if the vaccine strain poorly matches circulating influenza strains

Oseltamivir (oral) or zanamivir (inhaled) are the recommended anti-viral agents.

Preexposure

a. Influenza vaccine—there are several different formulations of the vaccine and methods of administration that are available.

Influenza vaccines—United States, 2015–2016 influenza season

- **Inactivated influenza vaccine, quadrivalent (IIV4), standard dose**
  - Fluarix Quadrivalent
  - FluLaval Quadrivalent
  - Fluzone Quadrivalent
  - Fluzone Intradermal Quadrivalent
- **Inactivated influenza vaccine, trivalent (IIV3), standard dose**
  - Afluria
  - Fluvirin
  - Fluzone
- **Inactivated influenza vaccine, trivalent (IIV3), high dose**
  - Fluzone High-Dose
- **Inactivated influenza vaccine, cell-culture-based (ccIIV3), standard dose**
  - Flucelvax
- **Recombinant influenza vaccine, trivalent (RIV3), standard dose**
  - FluBlok
- **Live, attenuated influenza vaccine, quadrivalent (LAIV4)**
    i. Quadrivalent inactivated influenza vaccine (IIV4)—given as IM injection to any person ≥ 6 months of age. The American Congress of Obstetrics and Gynecology (ACOG) strongly recommends that *all* women who will be pregnant during influenza season receive a dose of inactivated influenza vaccine—IIV4 or IIV3. The vaccine may be given during any trimester of pregnancy. Contraindication: severe

anaphylactic reaction to any vaccine component, including egg protein, or after previous dose of any influenza vaccine. Precautions: Moderate to severe acute illness with or without fever; history of Guillain-Barré syndrome within 6 weeks of receipt of influenza vaccine.

ii. Quadrivalent, intradermal influenza vaccine—given as an intradermal injection using a novel microinjection system. Vaccine is licensed for use in persons 18 to 64 years of age. Needle used is only 1.5 mm in length—injection system allows for reliable delivery of an accurate dose of antigen into dermal skin layer (2 mm). There is no need to alter the injection technique or needle length based on patient age, gender, muscle mass, or BMI. Contraindication: severe anaphylactic reaction to egg or egg products.

iii. Trivalent inactivated influenza vaccine (IIV3)—given as IM injection to any person ≥6 months of age. Contraindications and precautions the same as those for IIV4.

iv. Trivalent inactivated influenza vaccine (IIV3)—high-dose—given as IM injection—this vaccine that contains 4 times the amount of influenza antigen in standard dose influenza vaccine. It stimulates older individuals to produce higher levels of antibody and provides enhanced protection against influenza illness. It is associated with a higher risk of local injection site reactions but no higher risk of serious adverse events. This vaccine is recommended for persons aged ≥ 65 years.

v. Trivalent inactivated influenza vaccine, cell-culture-based (ccIIV3)—contraindications and precautions are the same as those for IIV3 and IIV4. It is not licensed for use in children <18 years of age.

vi. Trivalent recombinant influenza vaccine (RIV3)—this is the only influenza vaccine that is egg free. It is contraindicated in anyone with a history of a severe allergic reaction to any vaccine component, but safe for use in individuals with serious egg allergy. It is not licensed for use in children <18 years of age.

vii. Trivalent, intradermal influenza vaccine—given as an intradermal injection using a novel microinjection system. Vaccine is licensed for use in persons 18 to 64 years of age. Needle used is only 1.5 mm in length—injection system allows for reliable delivery of an accurate dose of antigen into dermal skin layer (2mm). There is no need to alter the injection technique or needle length based on patient age, gender, muscle mass, or BMI.

viii. Quadrivalent live attenuated, cold adapted influenza vaccine (LAIV)—given as a nasal spray. This vaccine is recommended only for healthy persons 2 to 49 years of age. Contraindications include: pregnancy, hives or anaphylaxis to egg or egg products, persons with known or suspected immunodeficiencies and children aged 2 through 4 years who have asthma or who have had a wheezing episode noted in the medical record within the past 12 months, or for whom parents report that a health-care provider stated that they had wheezing or asthma within the last 12 months.

Egg allergic patients

Egg allergy of any severity (including anaphylaxis) is no longer considered a contraindication or precaution to receiving injectable inactivated (IIV) or live, attenuated, intranasal (LAIV) influenza vaccines. Multiple published studies involving greater than 4,100 egg allergic patients (including those with severe anaphylactic reactions to egg) who have received IIV and over 1,200 egg allergic patients who have received LAIV have shown that these patients have tolerated the vaccines well with no hives or anaphylaxis. The CDC and the AAP Committee on Infectious Diseases have reviewed the data and feel that it supports that egg allergy does not impart an increased risk of anaphylactic reaction to immunization with either IIV or LAIV. Immediate hypersensitivity reactions such as urticarial or anaphylaxis may occur, however, these are no more common in egg-allergic than non-egg-allergic vaccine recipients. Anaphylactic reactions after influenza vaccine occur at the same rate as with other vaccines (about 1 per million persons vaccinated) whether the recipient is egg allergic or not and whether the vaccine contains egg or not. Special precautions regarding the medical setting and waiting period after administration of IIV or LAIV to egg allergic recipients beyond those recommended for any vaccine are not warranted. Persons with egg allergy of any severity can be safely vaccinated with IIV or LAIV in any setting.

Efficacy

The efficacy and effectiveness of influenza vaccines depend primarily on the age and immunocompetence of the vaccine recipients and the degree of similarity between the viruses in the vaccine and those circulating in the community. Efficacy in persons 2 years of age and older ranges from 50% to 95%. LAIV use was not recommended during the 2016–2017 influenza season because of low effectiveness during the 2013–2014 and 2014–2015 seasons.

Duration of protection

Duration of protection is 6 to 12 months—annual vaccination is critical to maintain protection against influenza in all populations.

Contraindications and precautions to influenza vaccines

Contraindications
- I. For inactivated, recombinant, and live, attenuated vaccines
  1. Severe allergic reaction (e.g., anaphylaxis) after previous dose of any influenza vaccine; or to a vaccine component
- II. Additional contraindications for live, attenuated vaccine
  1. Pregnant women
  2. Immunosuppressed persons
  3. Persons that have taken influenza antiviral medications (amantadine, rimantadine, zanamivir, or oseltamivir) within the previous 48 hours; avoid use of these antiviral drugs for 14 days after vaccination
  4. Asthma or a wheezing episode noted in the medical record within the past 12 months in children ages 2 through 4 years of age

Precautions
- I. For inactivated, recombinant, and live, attenuated vaccines

1. Moderate or severe acute illness with or without fever
2. History of Guillain-Barré syndrome within 6 weeks of previous influenza vaccination

II. Additional precautions for live, attenuated vaccine
1. Asthma in persons aged 5 years and older
2. Other chronic medical conditions such as other chronic lung disease, chronic cardiovascular disease (excluding isolated hypertension), diabetes, chronic renal or hepatic disease, hematologic disease, neurologic disease, and metabolic disorders

Frequently asked questions

What are the benefits of the flu vaccine?

Flu vaccination reduces the risk of influenza illness in recipients and protects those around recipients who may be more vulnerable to serious flu illness. Influenza vaccination also may make illness milder if someone does get sick and reduce the risk of more serious outcomes, like hospitalizations and deaths. Recent studies showed that flu vaccine reduced children's risk of flu-related pediatric intensive care unit (PICU) admission by 74% and flu-related hospitalizations among adults by 71% during the 2011–2012 flu season. Vaccination has been associated with lower rates of some cardiac events among people with heart disease, especially among those who had had a cardiac event in the past year.

Does protection from seasonal influenza vaccine decline several months after vaccination? Should I wait until flu season starts to vaccinate my elderly or medically frail patients?

Antibody to seasonal inactivated influenza vaccine does decline in the months following vaccination, but it should still be high enough to provide protection through the end of the season. Because the onset of flu season is unpredictable, seasonal influenza vaccine should be administered ideally by October. To avoid missed opportunities, offer vaccination during routine health care visits and hospitalizations when vaccine is available.

How long does immunity from seasonal influenza vaccine last?

Protection from influenza vaccine usually persists for about a year, although antibody persistence may be shorter for persons aged 65 and older. Vaccination is recommended on an annual basis because of waning antibody titers and because of changes in the circulating influenza viruses from year to year.

When should I stop offering influenza vaccination?

Continue to offer flu vaccine as long as influenza viruses are circulating in the community. The peak of influenza activity usually occurs in January or February in the United States. It is recommended that providers continue to vaccinate persons into the spring (typically through May).

If an unvaccinated patient has just recovered from a confirmed case of influenza, should that person be vaccinated with influenza vaccine?

Yes. Influenza vaccines contain 3 or 4 influenza strains, two influenza A strains, and one or two influenza B strains. Infection with one virus type does not confer immunity to other virus types and it is not unusual to be exposed to more than one strain during a typical influenza season. So a person who recently had influenza will benefit from a vaccine containing additional influenza virus strains.

Is Guillain-Barré syndrome an important risk for patients receiving influenza vaccination?

A significantly increased risk of GBS was reported in association with the swine flu vaccine in 1976. The reasons for that are unclear but since that time, the risk of GBS following flu vaccination has been estimated to be about 1 in 1,000,000 flu vaccine recipients. GBS is a risk following stimulation of the immune system whether by immunization or illness. Influenza illness is associated with a significantly greater risk of GBS than influenza vaccination, and the overall benefits of influenza vaccination far outweigh the risk of GBS.

Is influenza vaccine safe to administer to patients with multiple sclerosis?

Yes. Multiple sclerosis is not a contraindication to receiving any vaccine, including influenza vaccine. These patients should receive the inactivated influenza vaccine and not the live, attenuated influenza vaccine.

What type of influenza vaccine is recommended for pregnant women?

Pregnant women can receive any of the inactivated injectable vaccines. They should not be given the live, attenuated intransal influenza vaccine. It is important to vaccinate pregnant women during any trimester because of the increased risk of influenza-related complications, hospitalizations, and death. Vaccinating pregnant women protects the woman, her unborn baby, and the baby following birth from influenza disease.

What vaccine if any should I offer a patient with a history of egg allergy?
Persons able to eat a lightly cooked (e.g., scrambled) egg are unlikely to be allergic to eggs. Persons with a history of only hives can be offered inactivated influenza vaccine (IIV) with observation for at least 30 minutes for a reaction following administration or the egg-free preparation recombinant influenza vaccine (RIV) (Flublok). Those with a history of angioedema, respiratory distress, lightheadedness or recurrent emesis should be offered RIV. Persons with history of severe allergic reaction to flu vaccine should not receive flu vaccine again, regardless of the component suspected to be responsible for the reaction.

What is the value of high-dose flu vaccine?
High dose flu vaccine has been associated with significantly higher antibody responses and better protection against laboratory-confirmed influenza illness (24% efficacy in one large study) in persons ≥65 years.

What is the value of quadrivalent over trivalent influenza vaccines?
Quadrivalent flu vaccines cover an additional influenza B strain and should offer broader protection.

Who should not receive the live, attenuated influenza vaccine?
The following persons should not receive LAIV:

- children aged <2 years
- adults aged ≥50 years
- children aged 2 through 4 years with a wheezing episode during the preceding 12 months
- persons with asthma
- children and adults who have chronic pulmonary, cardio-vascular (except isolated hypertension), renal, hepatic, neurologic/neuromuscular, hematologic, or metabolic disorders
- immunosuppressed children and adults (including immu-nosuppression caused by medications or by HIV)
- pregnant women.

Patients will refuse influenza vaccination because they insist they "got the flu" after receiving the injectable vaccine in the past. How can I respond?

This misconception persists for several reasons: 1) Less than 1% of persons vaccinated with the injectable inactivated influenza vaccine develop flulike symptoms, such as mild fever and muscle aches after vaccination. These side effects are not the same as having influenza infection, but people commonly confuse the symptoms as being the same. 2) Protective immunity does not develop until 1 to 2 weeks after vaccination. Some people vaccinated later in the season may be infected with influenza virus shortly after receiving the vaccine before immunity is established. 3) Many people believe that "the flu" is any illness with fever and cold symptoms. If they get any viral respiratory illness, they blame it on the vaccine or believe that got "the flu" despite being vaccinated. Influenza vaccine protects against certain influenza viruses, not all viruses. 4) The influenza vaccine is not 100% effective, especially in older adults.

Can high-dose influenza vaccine be administered to patients younger than 65 years of age with chronic underlying conditions (e.g., HIV, immunodeficiency)?

No. The high-dose influenza vaccine is only licensed for persons aged 65 and older and is not recommended for younger persons with underlying medical conditions.

Can a person aged 65 or older who has already received a standard-dose influenza vaccine also receive a dose of high-dose influenza vaccine in the same influenza season?

No. It is not recommended that anyone receive more than one dose of influenza vaccine in the same season except for infants and children age 6 months to 8 years who are receiving influenza vaccine for the first time and for whom two doses of vaccine are recommended.

How soon after a bone marrow transplant can patients be vaccinated against influenza?

Inactivated influenza vaccine should be administered beginning 6 months after bone marrow transplant and annually thereafter.

Which health-care providers should be vaccinated against influenza?

It is important to vaccinate *all* hospital, outpatient, nursing home and chronic care facility health-care personnel with influenza vaccine, especially those that have direct patient contact. Vaccine response is diminished in elderly and immunosuppressed persons and evidence suggests vaccinating health-care personnel may be even more effective than vaccinating the patients themselves.

Which health-care personnel can receive the live, attenuated influenza vaccine (LAIV)?

LAIV can be administered to all healthcare personnel for whom it is indicated based on age and health history except those who care for severely immunocompromised patients in a protected (reverse air flow) environment.

If a patient is allergic to chicken or duck feathers is this a contraindication to receiving an egg-based influenza vaccine?

No.

Can LAIV be administered to persons with a mild upper respiratory infection with or without fever?

Yes, unless it is clinically deemed that the patient's nasal congestion would interfere with the delivery of the vaccine to the nasopharyngeal mucosa. In this case, administration of the vaccine should be deferred until the congestion resolves.

Can a woman who is breastfeeding receive LAIV?

Yes. Breastfeeding is not a contraindication for the receipt of any routine vaccine including LAIV. Postpartum maternal vaccination against influenza is associated with a significant reduction in illness, doctor visits and antibiotic prescriptions in infants during influenza season.

Can LAIV be given to contacts of immunosuppressed patients?

Household members, healthcare personnel and others with close contact to severely immunosuppressed individuals during periods in which the immunosuppressed person requires care in a protective environment should preferentially receive inactivated influenza vaccine.

What should be done in the situation when a young patient is only able to receive half the dose of the live attenuated intranasal vaccine (LAIV)?
A half dose of LAIV or any vaccine is a non-standard dose and should not be counted. If the second half of the dose is not administered at the same appointment, another full dose of influenza vaccine should be administered at another time. A dose of inactivated influenza vaccine can be administered at any time after the half dose of LAIV. If LAIV is given again, wait 4 weeks before administering another live vaccine.

What should be done is the situation when a patient believes they had a reaction to the influenza vaccine in the past and requests that the vaccine dose be split into 2 doses administered on different days?
This is not an acceptable practice. Doses of influenza vaccine or any other vaccine should not be split in half or partial doses. If a half or partial dose is administered, it is not counted as a valid dose and should be repeated as soon as possible with a full age-appropriate vaccine dose.

What should be done if a dose of intradermal influenza vaccine is administered to a patient that is not in the recommended age range of 18 to 64 years of age?
Persons younger than 12 years and older than 65 are more likely to have skin that is too thin for proper intradermal administration of the vaccine. A dose given to persons in these age ranges should be considered invalid and the patient should

be revaccinated with an age appropriate dose of vaccine. For person age 12 to 17 years, the dose can be considered valid and does not have to be repeated if the health-care provider is certain that the dose was administered intradermally and not subcutaneously. If there is any doubt whether the dose was injected intradermally, the dose should be repeated with an age-appropriate vaccine.

If a patient has already received a dose of seasonal trivalent influenza vaccine, is it acceptable to administer an additional dose of the quadrivalent influenza vaccine to this patient?
No, the CDC does not recommend more than one dose of influenza vaccine in a season, except for certain children ages 6 months through 8 years of age for whom two doses are recommended if this is the first season they are receiving influenza vaccine.

Which persons who are traveling abroad should influenza vaccine be given?
Health-care providers should vaccinate any person who failed to get vaccinated during the influenza season and who wants to reduce their risk of acquiring influenza during their travels. This includes persons who are traveling to the tropics, traveling with organized tourist groups at any time of the year or in the Southern Hemisphere from April through September.

If a patient received a dose of influenza vaccine in May for international travel, how long should the patient wait before getting vaccinated with the next season's influenza vaccine?
There should be a minimum of 4 weeks between the doses of influenza vaccine.

If a child needs 2 doses of influenza vaccine, can they receive 1 dose of injectable vaccine and 1 dose of the nasal spray vaccine?

Yes, as long as the child is eligible to receive nasal spray vaccine, it is acceptable to receive 1 dose of each type of influenza vaccine as long as the doses are spaced at least 4 weeks apart.

Can high dose influenza vaccine be administered to patients younger than 65 years of age with chronic underlying conditions (e.g., HIV, immunodeficiencies)?

No. The high dose influenza vaccine is only licensed for people age 65 years and older and is not recommended for younger persons with chronic underlying conditions.

Can a person age ≥65 years who has already received standard-dose influenza vaccine, also receive a dose of high dose influenza vaccine during the same influenza season?

No. It is not recommended that anyone receive more than one dose of influenza vaccine in the same season except for certain infants and children age 6 months through 8 years who are receiving influenza vaccine for the first time and for whom two doses are recommended.

If high dose influenza vaccine is not available, can 2 doses of standard-dose influenza vaccine be given to a person age ≥ 65 years in place of the high dose influenza vaccine?

No. This is not the same as high dose influenza vaccine and is not recommended.

REFERENCES

Des Roches A, Paradis L, Gagmon R, et al. Egg-allergic patients can be safely vaccinated against influenza. J Allergy Clin Immunol 2012;130:1213–1216.

The Joint Task Force on Practice Parameters. Update on influenza vaccination of egg allergic patients. Ann Allergy, Asthma & Immunol 2013;111:301–302.

Des Roches A, Samaan K, Graham F et al. Safe vaccination of patients with egg allergy by using live attenuated influenza vaccine. J Allergy Clin Immunol Pract 2015;3:138–139.

Turner PJ, Southern J, Andrews NJ, et al. Safety of live, attenuated influenza vaccine in atopic children with egg allergy. J Allergy Clin Immunol 2015;136:376–381.

Turner PJ, Southern J, Andrews NJ, et al. Safety of live, attenuated influenza vaccine in young people with egg allergy: multicenter prospective cohort study. BMJ 2015;351:h6291.

Kelso JM. Administering influenza vaccine to egg-allergic persons. Expert Rev Vaccines 2014;13:1049–1057.

HEPATITIS A

Did you know that:

- In 1988 an epidemic of hepatitis A in Shanghai, China, attributed to the consumption of raw clams affected 300,000 persons in a two-month period.
- Hepatitis A vaccination was first introduced in the United States in 1995, expanded to 17 "high-risk" states in 1999, and to all children aged 12 to 23 months of age in 2006. The incidence of hepatitis A has declined to an all-time low in recent years. The most susceptible population is now older adults in whom disease is typically more severe.

Hepatitis A virus is the cause of 20% to 40% of viral hepatitis cases in the Western world. The majority (over 70%) of cases in infants and children under 6 years of age are asymptomatic. Hepatitis A is the cause of an acute, self-limited illness associated with fever, malaise, jaundice, anorexia, and nausea that resolves in 2 months or less. Ten to 15% of symptomatic persons have prolonged or relapsing disease that may last as long as 6 months.

Hepatitis A infection in pregnancy may be associated with a high risk of maternal complications including: premature contractions, preterm labor, premature rupture of membranes, placental separation, vaginal bleeding, fetal distress and low birthweight infants.

Rates of hepatitis A in the United States are the lowest they have been in 40 years. The hepatitis A vaccine was introduced in 1995, and health professionals now routinely vaccinate all children, travelers to certain countries, and persons at risk for the disease. The use of hepatitis A vaccination has dramatically decreased rates of the disease in the United States (Figure 7).

Transmission:

1. Direct person to person contact via fecal-oral route
2. Ingestion of contaminated food or water
3. Oral or anal sex

Hepatitis A viruses persist in the environment and can withstand food-production processes routinely used to inactivate bacterial pathogens.

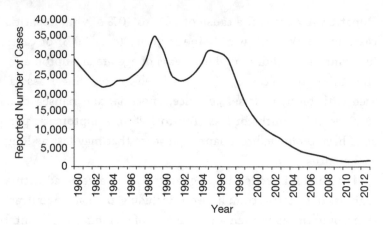

Figure 7 Incidence of hepatitis A, by year, United States, 1980–2013

Incubation period

Incubation period is on average 28 days (range: 15 to 50 days).

Prevention

Post-exposure

a. Administration of intramuscular immunoglobulin—if given within 2 weeks after exposure is greater than 85% effective in preventing symptomatic hepatitis A infection. Recommended to be administered to persons younger than 12 months of age, persons of any age who are immunocompromised or have chronic liver disease, and is preferred for persons 41 years of age and older.

b. Hepatitis A vaccine—if given within 2 weeks after exposure is greater than 85% effective in preventing symptomatic Hepatitis A infection. Recommended to be administered to persons 12 months through 40 years of age. May be used in persons 41 years of age and older if immunoglobulin not available.

Preexposure
   a. Hepatitis A vaccine—licensed for persons 12 months of age and older
   b. Immunoglobulin—persons younger than 12 months of age

Vaccine: Given intramuscularly as a 2 dose series at 0 and 12-18 months. Vaccine should not be given to those persons with hypersensitivity to any of the vaccine components.

Immunogenicity

95% after 1 dose, >99% after 2 doses

Duration of protection

At least 10 years after 2-dose series, but felt to be lifelong.

Contraindications and precautions to hepatitis A vaccine

Contraindications
   Severe allergic reaction (e.g., anaphylaxis) after a previous dose or to a vaccine component

Precautions
   Moderate or severe acute illness with or without fever

Frequently asked questions

How stable is hepatitis A virus (HAV) in the environment?

Depending on the environmental conditions, HAV can remain stable in the environment for months. Heating foods at temperatures greater than 185°F (85°C) for 1 minute or disinfecting surfaces with a 1:100 dilution of bleach in tap water will inactivate HAV.

Can people with HAV develop chronic disease?

Unlike hepatitis B and hepatitis C viruses, HAV does not cause chronic, long-term infection. Once you have had HAV infection and recover, you cannot get it again.

Should prevaccination testing be performed before administering Hepatitis A vaccine?

Prevaccination testing is recommended only in specific circumstances to reduce the costs of vaccinating people who are already immune to hepatitis A, including

- Persons born in geographic areas with high prevalence of HAV infection
- Older adolescents and adults in certain population groups (i.e., American Indians, Alaska Natives, and Hispanics)
- Adults in groups that have a high prevalence of infection (e.g., injection drug users)

Prevaccination testing might also be warranted for all older adults. The decision to test should be based on (1) the expected prevalence of immunity, (2) the cost of vaccination compared with the cost of serologic testing, and (3) the likelihood that testing will not interfere with vaccination.

Should postvaccination HAV titers be performed after a person has received the 2-dose vaccine series?
No. Postvaccination testing is *not* indicated because of the high rate of vaccine response among vaccine recipients. Also, not all testing methods approved for diagnostic use in the United States have the sensitivity to detect low, but protective, anti-HAV concentrations after vaccination.

Should health-care workers (HCWs) be routinely vaccinated against hepatitis A?
No. Studies have shown that HCWs are not at increased risk of HAV infection due to their occupation. The only HCWs for whom hepatitis A vaccine is routinely recommended are those who work with live HAV or with primates.

Should daycare workers be routinely vaccinated against hepatitis A?
No. Child care centers may be the source of outbreaks of hepatitis A in certain communities, HAV disease in child care centers more commonly reflects transmission from the community.

Can a breastfeeding woman receive hepatitis A vaccine?
Yes. Hepatitis A vaccine is an inactivated vaccine that poses no harm to the breastfeeding infant.

What should be done in the situation in which an adult patient inadvertently receives a dose of pediatric hepatitis A vaccine?
As a general rule, if a patient is given a vaccine dose that is less than a full age-appropriate dose of any vaccine, the dose

is invalid and the patient should be revaccinated with the age appropriate dose as soon as feasible. However, there are 2 exceptions to the general rule:

1. If a patient sneezes after receiving nasal spray live, attenuated influenza vaccine, the dose is counted as valid.
2. If an infant regurgitates, spits up, or vomits during or after receiving oral rotavirus vaccine, the dose is counted as valid.

If a patient receives more than an age-appropriate dose of a vaccine (e.g., infant receiving adult dose of HAV), the dose is counted as valid and caution must be taken not to repeat the error. Using larger than recommended doses can be hazardous because of excessive local or systemic concentrations of antigens or other vaccine constituents.

Can someone donate blood if they have had hepatitis A?
If a patient had hepatitis A before age 11 years of age, they may donate blood; if they were 11 years of age or older, they cannot donate blood.

When does protection from hepatitis A vaccine commence?
Protection begins approximately 2 to 4 weeks after the first vaccine dose. A second booster dose results in long-term protection.

Your patient is leaving for their trip abroad in a few days. Can they still get the hepatitis A vaccine?
The first dose of hepatitis A vaccine can be given at any time before departure and will provide some protection for most healthy people.

Who should receive post-exposure prophylaxis (PEP) after exposure to hepatitis A?

People who might benefit from PEP include those who:

- Live with someone who has hepatitis A
- Have recently had sexual contact with someone who has hepatitis A
- Have recently shared injection or non-injection illegal drugs with someone who has hepatitis A
- Have had ongoing, close personal contact with a person with hepatitis A, such as a regular babysitter or caregiver
- Have been exposed to food or water known to be contaminated with HAV

Is it harmful to administer an extra dose(s) of hepatitis A vaccine or to repeat the entire vaccine series if documentation of vaccination history is unavailable?

No. If necessary, administering extra doses of hepatitis A vaccine is not harmful.

What are the current CDC guidelines for post-exposure protection against Hepatitis A?

Persons who have recently been exposed to HAV and who have not been vaccinated previously should be administered a single dose of hepatitis A vaccine or IG (0.02 mL/kg) as soon as possible and within 2 weeks after exposure.

- For healthy persons aged 12 months to 40 years, hepatitis A vaccine is preferred to IG because of the vaccine's advantages (long-term protection, ease of administration, and equivalent efficacy).
- For persons aged 40 years and older, IG is preferred because of the absence of data regarding vaccine performance in

this age group and because of the more severe manifestations of hepatitis A in older adults.

- Vaccine can be used if IG cannot be obtained.
- IG should be used for children aged less than 12 months, immunocompromised persons, persons with chronic liver disease, and persons who are allergic to the vaccine.

HEPATITIS B

Did you know that:

- Despite the availability of an effective vaccine, worldwide, hepatitis B virus (HBV) infection kills a person every 30 to 45 seconds.
- HBV is 100 times more infectious than HIV.
- An estimated 350 million people worldwide are chronically infected with HBV and 15% to 40% will develop severe serious sequelae (e.g., cirrhosis, liver failure, and hepatocellular carcinoma) during their lifetime.

There are an estimated 46,000 new cases of hepatitis B virus (HBV) infection reported each year in the United States; however, the CDC recognizes that this only accounts for 10% of the cases. Adults 30 to 49 years of age account for the majority of the new cases being reported. Hepatitis B infection accounts for 2,000 to 4,000 deaths each year primarily due to cirrhosis and liver cancer. The likelihood of developing symptoms of acute hepatitis is age dependent: <1% of infants younger than 1 year of age, 5% to 15% of children 1 to 5 years of age, and 30% to 50% of people older than 5 years of age are symptomatic. The spectrum of signs and symptoms includes subacute illness with nonspecific symptoms (e.g., anorexia, nausea, or malaise), clinical hepatitis with jaundice, or fulminant hepatitis, and extrahepatic manifestations such as arthralgia, arthritis, macular rashes, thrombocytopenia, polyarteritis nodosa, glomerulonephritis, or papular acrodermatitis (Gianotti-Crosti syndrome).

Risk factors for hepatitis B infection include:

- Travelers to countries where HBV infection is highly endemic
- Persons adopting or fostering children from countries where HBV infection is highly endemic
- Household contacts and sexual partners of person with HBV acute infection or chronic carriers
- Tattooing, piercing, or other forms of body modification
- Health-care, public safety workers exposed to blood and other fluids
- Staff and patients of institutions for the developmentally disabled, assisted-living facilities, and nursing homes
- Correctional facilities
- Persons with end stage renal disease, chronic liver disease, DM, HIV, or hemodialysis patients
- Men who have sex with men
- Persons seeking evaluation or treatment for a sexually transmitted infection especially HIV and syphilis
- Current or recent injection-drug users
- Sexually active persons with multiple sexual partners

60% of persons infected with HBV *do not* have an identifiable risk factor.

Age at time of acute infection is the primary determinant of the risk of progression to chronic infection.

- Risk is 5% if HBV infection is acquired as an adult.
- Risk is 30% to 50% if the infection is acquired as a child <5 years of age.
- Risk is >90% if infection is acquired as neonate.

Transmission

Hepatitis B is transmitted through percutaneous and permucosal exposure to infected blood and body fluids (including serum, semen, vaginal secretions, CSF, synovial, pleural, pericardial, peritoneal, and amniotic fluids) with serum, semen, vaginal secretions, and amniotic fluid being the most infectious. The most common modes of transmission are parenteral, sexual, and perinatal.

Incubation period

Incubation period is on average 90 days (range 45 to 160 days).

Hepatitis B and pregnancy

Women who are pregnant and have an acute hepatitis B infection are at increased risk for having a premature or low birthweight infant. Universal screening of *all* pregnant women for HBsAg, regardless of HBV vaccination history, is strongly recommended and should be performed during an early prenatal visit with every pregnancy. Perinatal transmission poses an extremely high risk to the infant for developing chronic disease and its complications. There are an estimated 20,000 infants each year born to women known to be infected with HBV infection (remember that only 10% of cases in adults are reported so that vast majority of cases are unrecognized). Perinatal transmission of HBV is highly efficient and usually occurs from blood exposure during labor and delivery. In the absence of post-exposure treatment, 6,000 of the 20,000 infants would develop chronic infection, and 25% will die prematurely from HBV-related hepatocellular carcinoma or cirrhosis.

If a mother is HBsAg positive at time of delivery, 20% of infants born to these mothers will be infected with HBV—in the absence of post-exposure treatment, 90% of these infants will go on to become chronic carriers.

If a mother is HBsAg positive *and* HBeAg positive (marker for transmissibility—very high viral loads) at the time of delivery, 70% to 90% of infants born to these mothers will be infected with HBV—in the absence of post-exposure treatment, >90% of these infants will go on to become chronic carriers.

Prevention

Postexposure

a. Perinatal—hepatitis B immune globulin (HBIG) given within 12 hours of birth *and* a dose of HBV vaccine—use of this regimen is 95% effective in preventing transmission of HBV to infant. Standard immune globulin (IG) is *not* effective for postexposure prophylaxis against HBV infection because concentrations of hepatitis B antibodies are too low.

b. Discrete exposure to an HBsAg-positive source (e.g., percutaneous—needlestick, bite, nonintact skin or mucosal exposure to HBsAg positive blood or body fluids; sexual contact or needle sharing with HBsAg positive person; victim of sexual assault/abuse by a person who is HBsAg positive)—HBIG and hepatitis B vaccine to complete series

c. Household contact of HBsAg positive person or exposure to a source with unknown HBsAg status—administer hepatitis B vaccine series

Preexposure
> Administer hepatitis B vaccine series—given intramuscularly
> as 3-dose series at 0, 1, and 6 month intervals.

Vaccine efficacy

Efficacy is 90% to 95% after 3 doses for preventing HBV infection and clinical HBV disease.

Duration of protection

At least 20 years but probably lifelong. Confers protection against clinical illness and chronic HBV infection.

Vaccine contraindications and precautions

Contraindications
> Severe allergic reaction (e.g., anaphylaxis) after a previous
> dose or to a vaccine component.

Precautions
> Moderate or severe acute illness with or without fever

Frequently asked questions

Can hepatitis B virus (HBV) be transmitted in the daycare setting by the saliva of drooling infants?
HBV has been found in saliva, but there is no data indicating that saliva exposure alone can transmit a HBV infection. If a HBV-infected person bites another person, HBV can be transmitted; however, it is the blood in the infected person's mouth from the bite that was the likely vehicle of transmission. HBV

is not spread by casual contact, sneezing, kissing, coughing, sharing eating utensils or drinking containers, or by food or water.

Can a patient who had an acute hepatitis B infection that was completely resolved ever get hepatitis B infection again?

In general, the answer is no. However, it is possible for this person to acquire a different HBV variant or subtype as the cause of the second infection. This would be a very rare occurrence.

I run a clinic for patients who are chronic hepatitis B carriers. How stable is HBV in the environment, and what type of disinfectant should I use to clean my waiting room and exam rooms?

HBV is very stable in the environment and remains viable for 7 or more days on environmental surfaces at room temperature. It is capable of transmitting HBV infection despite the absence of visible blood. Any disinfectant that is tuberculocidal will kill HBV.

What screening blood test should be done in pregnant women to prevent perinatal HBV infection?

Screening should be done with the hepatitis B surface antigen (HBsAg) test only. This test will determine whether a woman currently has a HBV infection that she can transmit to her infant. Other HBV tests such as antibody to hepatitis B core antigen (anti-HBc) and hepatitis B surface antibody (anti-HBs) are not useful when screening to prevent perinatal HBV infections and should not be used in the screening process.

If a woman has been previously vaccinated against HBV infection does she still need to screened for HBV during pregnancy?

Yes. Women who have received hepatitis B vaccine should still be screened for HBsAg early in each pregnancy. Just because she is vaccinated does not mean that she is HBsAg negative.

Can a pregnant woman receive hepatitis B vaccine?

Yes. Current hepatitis B vaccines contain noninfectious HBsAg and pose no risk to the developing fetus.

How should an infant be managed if their mother's HBsAg test result is not available at the time of birth?

1. Women without documentation of HBsAg test results at the time of admission for delivery should have blood drawn and tested as soon as possible after admission.

2. All infants born to women without documentation of HBsAg test results should receive the first dose of single-antigen hepatitis B vaccine (without HBIG) by 12 hours of age.

3. If the mother is found to be HBsAg positive, her infant should receive HBIG as soon as possible but no later than 7 days of age, and the HBV vaccine series should be completed according to the recommended schedule for infants born to HBsAg positive mothers.

4. If the mother is found to be HBsAg negative, the infant's HBV vaccine series should be completed according to the recommended schedule.

Is it safe for an HBsAg positive mother to breastfeed her infant?

Yes. An HBsAg positive mother should be encouraged to breastfeed her infant if she wishes to do so. The infant should receive HBIG and hepatitis B vaccine within 12 hours of birth. Even though HBV can be detected in breast milk, studies have shown that breastfed infants born to HBsAg positive mothers do not have an increased rate of perinatal or early childhood HBV infection.

What should be done in the situation where an infant inadvertently receives a dose of the adult formulation of hepatitis B vaccine?
The adult formation of hepatitis B vaccine contains twice the amount of antigen compared to a dose of the infant/child formulation. If an infant receives an adult dose of the hepatitis B vaccine, the dose is counted as valid and does not need to be repeated. Hepatitis B vaccine is a very safe vaccine and no adverse events would be expected. The next age appropriate dose should be given on the routine schedule.

Is post-vaccination serologic testing recommended for adults who receive hepatitis B vaccine?
Testing is not necessary after routine vaccination of adults. Serologic testing for immunity after vaccination is recommended only for people whose subsequent clinical management depends on knowledge of their immune status. Post-vaccination testing is recommended for: health-care and public safety workers at increased risk for continued exposure to blood on the job; immune compromised individuals; and sex and needle sharing partners of HBsAg positive persons. Testing should be performed 1 to 2 months after the last dose of vaccine. However, CDC does not recommend routine testing of health-care personnel who were not tested within the 1- to 2-month postvaccination time period. Health-care

personnel who are exposed to HBV can be tested as part of postexposure management.

What should be done in the situation where a person has received an appropriate 3-dose series of HBV vaccine but their anti-HBs (HBsAb) titer is negative (less than 10 mIU/mL)?
Repeat the 3-dose HBV vaccine series, and the person should be tested for anti-HBs 1 to 2 months after the third dose of the vaccine. If the anti-HBs test is still negative after the second vaccine series, the person should be tested for HBsAg and anti-HBc to determine their HBV infection status. People who test negative for HBsAg and anti-HBc should be considered vaccine non-responders and susceptible to HBV infection. These patients should be counseled about precautions to prevent HBV infection and the need to obtain hepatitis B immunoglobulin (HBIG) prophylaxis for any known or likely exposure to HBsAg-positive blood. Persons found to be HBsAg negative but anti-HBc positive were infected in the past and require no vaccination or treatment.

MEASLES

Did you know that:

- The 7-year-old daughter of Roald Dahl, the British author of *Charlie and the Chocolate Factory*, died from a measles infection in 1962, the year before a measles vaccine became available. Dahl went on to become a strong supporter of vaccines: "In my opinion parents who now refuse to have their children immunized are putting the lives of

those children at risk. In America, where measles immunization is compulsory, measles like smallpox, has been
virtually wiped out. Here in Britain, because so many parents refuse, either out of obstinacy or ignorance or fear, to
allow their children to be immunized, we still have a hun-
dred thousand cases of measles every year."

- Currently on a worldwide basis, 13 people die from measles every hour; measles continues to kill 430 children
each day.

Measles virus causes an acute viral illness characterized by fever,
cough, conjunctivitis, coryza, pharyngitis, erythematous maculopapular rash (starts on forehead around hairline and spreads
centrifugally from the head to the feet, becoming confluent),
lymphadenopathy (cervical, suboccipital and postauricular), and
Koplik spots (white lesions on an erythematous base on buccal
mucosa opposite the lower molars). It is one of the most contagious viral infections with secondary attack rates of over 90% in
susceptible household contacts.

Complications

Complications include otitis media; diarrhea; bronchopneumo-
nia (responsible for 60% of deaths associated with measles disease and may be measles virus associated and/or a secondary
bacterial superinfection with *Streptococcus pneumoniae*, group
A *Streptococcus, Staphylococcus aureus*); acute encephalitis (more
common in adults, associated with fever, headache, seizures,
altered consciousness, permanent neurologic sequelae and brain
damage); and subacute sclerosing panencephalitis (SSPE). SSPE
is a rare degenerative central nervous disease that occurs 7 to

10 years after wild-type measles infection, especially in those who had measles before 2 years of age. It is caused by a persistent infection with a mutant measles related virus in the CNS. It is characterized by behavioral and intellectual deterioration and seizures.

Measles infection during pregnancy maybe associated with a risk of miscarriage and prematurity. Pneumonia (both measles virus associated and secondary bacterial superinfection) is a major complication in pregnant women with measles.

Significant declines in measles vaccination rates or lack of measles vaccination in various areas of the world have resulted in a major resurgence in endemic disease. In 2011, France had the highest number of measles cases in the world. Many countries in Europe, Asia, Africa, South America, and New Zealand are also experiencing large numbers of measles cases. The majority of the cases seen in the United States are brought in by infected persons from other countries or by unvaccinated persons who contract the disease while traveling to countries where measles is endemic.

Transmission

The disease is transmitted person to person by direct contact with droplets from infected respiratory secretions. Persons are contagious from 4 days before the rash to 4 days after appearance of the rash.

Incubation period

8 to 12 days.

Prevention

Post-exposure

a. Administration of immunoglobulin can be given to prevent or modify measles in a susceptible person within 6 days of exposure. It is indicated for susceptible household or other close contacts of persons with measles, particularly contacts under 1 year of age, pregnant women, and immunocompromised people, for whom the risk of complications is highest, or in those persons in whom measles vaccine is contraindicated.

b. MMR (measles, mumps, rubella) vaccine, if given within 72 hours of measles exposure, will provide protection in some cases.

Preexposure

a. MMR vaccine—live, attenuated vaccine containing measles, mumps, and rubella viruses. Recommended for use in persons born in 1957 or later with first dose given to those 12 months of age and older.

b. Given subcutaneously (SQ) as MMR vaccine as a 2-dose series with minimal interval of 28 days between doses. In infants first dose is given at 12 to 15 months of age with second dose given at 4 to 6 years of age.

c. Inadvertent administration of MMR vaccine to a pregnant woman is *not* an indication for termination of the pregnancy.

Immunogenicity

95% after 1 dose, >99% after 2 doses

Duration of protection

Lifelong after 2 doses

Contraindications and precautions for MMR vaccine

Contraindications

1. History of severe (anaphylactic) reaction to neomycin (or other vaccine component) or following a previous dose of MMR
2. Pregnancy
3. Severe immunosuppression from either disease or therapy

Precautions

1. Receipt of an antibody-containing blood product in the previous 11 months
2. Moderate or severe acute illness with or without fever
3. History of thrombocytopenia or thrombocytopenic purpura

Frequently asked questions

Why does being born before 1957 confer immunity to measles?

People born before 1957 lived through a number of years of epidemic measles before the first measles vaccine was licensed in 1963. Because of this, these people are very likely to have had measles disease. Data from survey studies suggest that 95% to 98% of those born before 1957 are immune to measles. However, if serologic testing indicates that the person is not immune, at least 1 dose of MMR should be administered.

What are the current CDC criteria for evidence of immunity to measles, mumps, and rubella?

The current CDC criteria for evidence of immunity to measles, mumps, and rubella are:

1. Documented receipt to two appropriately timed doses of MMR vaccine, the first dose of which was given after 1 year of age
2. Laboratory confirmation of disease
3. Born before 1957

Physician diagnosis of disease has been removed as reliable evidence of immunity.

What should be done in the situation in which the MMR vaccine was given intramuscularly (IM) instead of subcutaneously (SC)?

It is recommended that all live injected vaccines (e.g., MMR, varicella, and yellow fever) be given SC; however, IM administration of these vaccines does not decrease immunogenicity and doses given IM do *not* need to be repeated.

What should be done in the situation in which MMRV vaccine was mistakenly given to an adult instead of MMR?

MMRV vaccine is licensed for use in persons 1 year to 12 years of age. If it is given to a patient 13 years of age and older it is considered to be off-label use. This dose may be counted as valid toward the completion of the MMR and varicella vaccine series and does not need to be repeated.

What are the current CDC recommendations for the administration of a dose of MMR vaccine to infants 6 to 11 months of age who will be traveling internationally?

CDC recommends that children who will be traveling or living abroad should be vaccinated with MMR vaccine at an earlier age than that recommended for children who live in the United States given that the risk for measles exposure can be high in both developed and developing countries. It is recommended that children age 6 to 11 months receive 1 dose of MMR vaccine before departure from the United States. This dose does not count toward the 2 recommended doses of MMR at 12 to 15 months and 4 to 6 years.

Can MMR vaccine be given to a child whose sibling is receiving chemotherapy?

Yes. MMR and varicella vaccines should be given to the healthy household contacts of immunosuppressed patients.

Is egg allergy considered a contraindication to receiving MMR vaccine?

No. Studies have documented the safety of giving MMR vaccine (which is grown in chick embryo tissue culture) to children with severe egg allergy. Egg allergy is *not* considered a contraindication to MMR vaccine, and the CDC and AAP recommend routine MMR vaccination of egg-allergic children without the use of special protocols or desensitization procedures.

Can MMR vaccine be given to a breastfeeding mother or to a breastfed infant?

Yes, breastfeeding does not interfere with the response to MMR vaccine and vaccination of a woman who is breastfeeding poses no risk to the infant being breastfed.

MUMPS

Did you know that:

- The clinical picture of mumps (*swelling about one or both ears and, in some instances, painful swelling of one or both testes...*) was first described by Hippocrates in the 5th century BC in Book 1 of his Book of Epidemics.
- Orchitis, an inflammation of the testicles, occurs in approximately 25% of males that are infected with mumps after puberty, up to 50% of those affected develop testicular atrophy, and 10% will have a drop in their sperm count.

Mumps is a systemic disease characterized most commonly by swelling of one or more of the salivary glands, usually the parotid glands. About one-third of the infections do not have clinically apparent salivary gland swelling and may be asymptomatic or manifest primarily as a respiratory tract infection. Infection in adults is much more likely to result in complications.

Complications

Over 50% of people with mumps have cerebrospinal fluid pleocytosis, but less than 10% have symptoms of viral meningitis. Symptoms are most commonly seen in older children, adolescents, and adults. Epididymo-orchitis is a common complication reported in 15% to 40% of post-pubertal males, especially in persons in the second, third, and fourth decades of life. It is usually unilateral but may be bilateral in up to 30% of cases. Oophoritis occurs in 7% of post-pubertal females. The incidence of deafness as a complication is 0.5 to 5 per 100,000 cases; it is usually unilateral and permanent.

Mumps infection during pregnancy is associated with increased rates of fetal mortality in women who contract mumps during the first trimester of pregnancy (27.3% vs. 13% in healthy controls). Even though mumps virus can cross the placenta, this mortality is not associated with the development of fetal malformations. Other complications in pregnant women include: mastitis, aseptic meningitis, and glomerulonephritis.

Large outbreaks have been seen in recent years on college campuses, among the Hasidic Jewish communities in New York and New Jersey, and among professional sports teams.

Transmission

Contact with infectious respiratory tract secretions and saliva. The period of maximum communicability is several days before and after the onset of parotid swelling.

Incubation period

16 to 18 days

Prevention

Post-exposure
   a. Immunoglobulin preparations are *not* effective as post-exposure prophylaxis for mumps.
   b. MMR (measles, mumps, rubella) vaccine has *not* been demonstrated to be effective in preventing infection after exposure. MMR vaccine can be given after exposure, because immunization will provide protection against subsequent exposures.

Preexposure

    a. MMR vaccine—live, attenuated vaccine containing measles, mumps, and rubella viruses. Recommended for use in persons born in 1957 or later with first dose given to those 12 months of age and older.

    b. Given subcutaneously as MMR vaccine as a 2-dose series with minimal interval of 28 days between doses. In infants first dose is given at 12 to 15 months of age with second dose given at 4 to 6 years of age. Inadvertent administration of MMR vaccine to a pregnant woman is *not* an indication for termination of the pregnancy.

Immunogenicity

73% to 91% after 1 dose, 79% to 95% after 2 doses

Duration of protection

Lifelong after 2 doses

Contraindications and precautions for MMR vaccine

Contraindications

    1. History of severe (anaphylactic) reaction to neomycin (or other vaccine component) or following a previous dose of MMR

    2. Pregnancy

    3. Severe immunosuppression from either disease or therapy. This includes people with conditions such as congenital immunodeficiency, AIDS, leukemia, lymphoma, generalized malignancy, and those receiving treatment for cancer with drugs, radiation, or large doses of corticosteroids.

Precautions

1. Receipt of an antibody-containing blood product in the previous 11 months
2. Moderate or severe acute illness with or without fever
3. History of thrombocytopenia or thrombocytopenic purpura

Frequently asked questions

How long is a person with mumps contagious?

People with mumps are considered most infectious from a few days before until 5 days after the onset of parotitis (facial swelling). The CDC recommends isolating mumps patients for 5 days after their glands begin to swell.

Can someone who had a laboratory confirmed case of mumps get mumps again?

People who have had mumps are usually protected for life against another mumps infection. However, second occurrences of mumps do rarely happen.

Which adult patients should receive 2 doses of MMR vaccine?

Certain adults are at higher risk of exposure to measles, mumps, and/or rubella and should receive a second dose of MMR unless they have other evidence of immunity; this includes adults who are

- Students in postsecondary educational institutions
- Health-care personnel
- Living in a community experiencing an outbreak or recently exposed to the disease

- Planning to travel internationally (for measles and mumps)
- People who received inactivated (killed) measles vaccine or measles vaccine of unknown type during the period 1963 to 1967 should be revaccinated with two doses of MMR vaccine.
- People vaccinated before 1979 with either killed mumps vaccine or mumps vaccine of unknown type who are at high risk for mumps infection (e.g., people who are working in a health-care facility) should be considered for revaccination with 2 doses of MMR vaccine.

RUBELLA

Did you know that:

- Rubella, first described in the late 18th century as a mild exanthematous disease of children and young adults, exploded onto the world stage when it was recognized in 1941 that it was a prominent cause of congenital defects in the fetus after maternal infection during pregnancy.
- The sweat of patients with rubella smells like freshly plucked chicken feathers.

Rubella (German measles) is caused by Rubella virus. The majority of postnatal rubella cases are subclinical and asymptomatic. Clinical disease is mild and characterized by a generalized erythematous maculopapular rash, lymphadenopathy, and low grade fever. The rash starts on the face, becomes generalized over 24 hours, and lasts a median of 3 days. Lymphadenopathy, which may precede the rash, often involves the posterior auricular or suboccipital lymph nodes but can be generalized, and lasts between 5 and 8 days. Transient polyarthralgia and polyarthritis are commonly seen in adolescents and adults, especially females. Due to the success of the vaccination program, the rubella cases seen in the United States occur in persons born in other countries who were never vaccinated or in underimmunized people.

Complications

Encephalitis (1 in 6,000 cases) and thrombocytopenia (1 in 3,000 cases).

Rubella during pregnancy is associated with a higher incidence of miscarriage, fetal death, or the congenital rubella syndrome (a constellation of congenital anomalies). The most common clinical manifestations seen in the infant at the time of birth include: "blueberry muffin" lesions (erythropoiesis in dermis and upper subcutaneous adipose tissue), growth restriction, interstitial pneumonitis, hepatosplenomegaly, thrombocytopenia, and radiolucent bone lesions. The most common anomalies associated with the congenital rubella syndrome are: ophthalmologic (cataracts, microphthalmia, and congenital glaucoma); cardiac (patent ductus arteriosus, peripheral pulmonary artery stenosis); auditory (sensorineural hearing loss); and neurologic (meningoencephalitis, microcephaly, mental retardation).

Congenital defects occur in up to 85% of cases if maternal infection occurs during the first 12 weeks of gestation, 50% during the first 13 to 16 weeks of gestation, and 25% during the end of the second trimester.

Transmission

Direct or droplet contact from infected nasopharyngeal secretions. The period of maximal communicability occurs from a few days before to 7 days after the onset of rash.

Incubation period

16 to 18 days

Prevention

Post-exposure

a. Immunoglobulin preparations are *not* effective as post-exposure prophylaxis for rubella and is *not* recommended for routine post-exposure prophylaxis of rubella in early pregnancy or any other circumstance.

b. MMR (measles, mumps, rubella) vaccine has *not* been demonstrated to be effective in preventing infection after exposure. MMR vaccine can be given after exposure, because immunization will provide protection against subsequent exposures.

Post-exposure evaluation of the pregnant woman includes:

a. Obtaining a blood sample as soon as possible after exposure and testing for rubella IgM and IgG antibodies. An aliquot of frozen serum should be stored for possible repeated testing at a later time. The presence of rubella-specific IgG antibody at the time of exposure indicates that the person is most likely immune.

b. If antibody is not detectable, a second blood specimen should be obtained 2 to 3 weeks later and tested concurrently with the first specimen.

c. If the second test result is negative, another blood specimen should be obtained 6 weeks after the exposure and also tested concurrently with the first specimen.

d. A **negative test result** in **both the second and third specimens** indicates that infection has *not* occurred.

e. A **positive test result** in the **second or third specimen** but *not* the **first** indicates a **recent** infection.

Preexposure
a. MMR vaccine—live, attenuated vaccine containing measles, mumps and rubella viruses. Recommended for use in persons born in 1957 or later with first dose given to those 12 months of age and older. Contraindictated in persons who are pregnant, persons with certain immunodeficiencies or those who had a previous anaphylactic reaction to the vaccine or any of its components.

Vaccine: Given subcutaneously as MMR vaccine as a 2-dose series with minimal interval of 28 days between doses. In infants first dose is given at 12 to 15 months of age with second dose given at 4 to 6 years of age. Inadvertent administration of MMR vaccine to a pregnant woman is *not* an indication for termination of the pregnancy.

Immunogenicity

73% to 91% after 1 dose, 79% to 95% after 2 doses

Duration of protection

Lifelong after 2 doses

Contraindications and precautions for MMR vaccine

Contraindications
1. History of severe (anaphylactic) reaction to neomycin (or other vaccine component) or following a previous dose of MMR.

2. Pregnancy
3. Severe immunosuppression from either disease or therapy

Precautions

1. Receipt of an antibody-containing blood product in the previous 11 months
2. Moderate or severe acute illness with or without fever
3. History of thrombocytopenia or thrombocytopenic purpura

Frequently asked questions

What is the recommended length of time a woman should wait after receiving MMR (rubella) vaccine before becoming pregnant?
CDC recommends deferring pregnancy for 4 weeks after receiving MMR vaccine.

What should be done in the situation in which a pregnant woman inadvertently was given an MMR vaccine?
MMR vaccination during pregnancy alone is not a reason to terminate the pregnancy. No specific action needs to be taken other than to reassure the woman that no adverse outcomes are expected as a result of this vaccination.

What should be done in the situation in which a pregnant woman's rubella test result shows that she is "not immune" but she has documentation of receiving 2 appropriately timed doses of MMR vaccine?
It is now recommended that women of childbearing age who have received 1 or 2 doses of a rubella-containing vaccine and have serum rubella IgG titers that are not positive should be

administered 1 additional dose of MMR vaccine (maximum 3 doses) and do not need to be retested for serologic evidence of rubella immunity. MMR vaccine should not be administered to a pregnant woman. The dose should be given after the baby is delivered.

How soon after delivery can MMR vaccine be given?
MMR vaccine may be administered any time after delivery. It should be administered before hospital discharge, even if the patient has received RhoGam during the hospital stay, is discharged in less than 24 hours, or is breastfeeding.

Is there any evidence that MMR vaccine or thimerosal are causes of autism spectrum disorder (ASD)?
NO. This is an issue that has been studied extensively, including several thorough reviews by the Institute of Medicine (IOM). A 2004 scientific review by the IOM concluded that "the evidence favors rejection of a causal relationship between thimerosal–containing vaccines and ASD." Since 2003, there have been nine CDC-funded or conducted studies that have found no link between thimerosal-containing vaccines and ASD, as well as no link between the measles, mumps, and rubella (MMR) vaccine and ASD in children. In 2011 an IOM report on eight routinely used vaccines (MMR, hepatitis A, meningococcal, varicella zoster, influenza, hepatitis B, HPV, and tetanus-containing vaccines) given to children and adults found that these vaccines are very safe and that there is no link between receiving vaccines and developing ASD. A 2013 CDC study added to the research showing that vaccines do not cause ASD. The study looked at the number of antigens (substances in vaccines that cause the body's immune system to produce disease-fighting antibodies) from vaccines

during the first two years of life. The results showed that the total amount of antigen from vaccines received was the same between children with ASD and those that did not have ASD. All the extensive research performed to date shows absolutely no evidence of any link between receiving vaccines or those vaccines containing trace thimerosal and ASD.

How likely is it for a person to develop arthritis after receiving an MMR vaccine?
Joint pain or arthralgia and transient arthritis following MMR vaccination occurs only in people who were susceptible to rubella at the time of vaccination. About 25% of non-immune post-pubertal women report joint pain after receiving a rubella-containing vaccine, and about 10% to 30% report arthritis-like signs and symptoms. If joint symptoms occur, it is generally 1 to 3 weeks after vaccination, are mild and last about 2 days.

How soon must MMR vaccine be administered once it has been reconstituted with diluent?
Optimally MMR vaccine should be administered immediately after reconstitution. If reconstituted, MMR vaccine should be used within 8 hours. If it is not used within this time period it should be discarded. The dose should be refrigerated and should never be left at room temperature.

VARICELLA ZOSTER (CHICKENPOX)

Did you know that:

- In 2011 in a misguided attempt to expose their children to the chickenpox virus to build immunity later in life, a group of parents across the United States (Tennessee, Arizona, California) started trading chickenpox virus-laced lollipops by mail, which is a federal crime.

- Prior to the introduction of varicella vaccine, varicella accounted for 10,600 hospitalizations and 100 to 150 deaths each year in the United States. That equates to 1 to 2 deaths each week!
- Primary varicella infection (chicken pox) wasn't differentiated from smallpox until the end of the 18th century.

Primary infection with **varicella zoster virus (VZV)** results in varicella (chickenpox). VZV establishes latency in the dorsal root ganglia after primary infection and reactivation at a later time results in herpes zoster (shingles). Varicella is a highly contagious disease with an 80% to 100% secondary household attack rate in unvaccinated persons. The appearance of the rash is preceded by a 1 to 2 day prodrome of fever, malaise, headache, and abdominal pain. The rash appears as crops of lesions that develop over several days. Each crop progresses within 24 hours from macules to papules to vesicles, and then pustules before crusting. All lesions are on an erythematous base and are pruritic. Lesions are in different stages of development at any given time and classically are described as "dew drops on a rose petal". The rash usually starts on the face and trunk and then spreads to the extremities and all other areas of the body. Usually between 250 and 500 lesions develop and all lesions are usually crusted by 4 to 7 days after onset of the rash. Recovery from primary varicella usually results in lifetime immunity. In otherwise healthy persons a second occurrence of varicella is uncommon but it can happen.

Complications include secondary bacterial infections of the skin lesions most commonly caused by group A *Streptococcus* and *Staphylococcus aureus* (which may progress to necrotizing fasciitis); pneumonia(viral or bacterial) which occurs in 15% of adults and is the most common complication in this population; central nervous system manifestations (e.g., cerebellar ataxia, meningoencephalitis, encephalitis); hepatitis; thrombocytopenia; acute respiratory distress syndrome; and hemorrhagic complications.

Persons at the highest risk of complications of varicella include: healthy adults, pregnant women, developing fetuses, infants born to mothers who have varicella five days before and 2 days after the delivery, and immunocompromised persons of any age. The risk of varicella complications is 10 to 20 times higher in adults than in children.

Congenital varicella syndrome (fetal varicella syndrome) may occur in women with maternal varicella infection occurring during the first two trimesters of pregnancy. There is an estimated 2% incidence of congenital disease after maternal varicella infection when occurring in the first 20 weeks' gestation. Characteristic features in affected infants include: low birthweight; skin lesions or scarring in a dermatomal distribution (76%); neurologic defects (e.g., microcephaly) (60% of cases); ophthalmologic disease (51%), and skeletal anomalies (e.g., hypoplasia of the extremities), muscle atrophy (50% of cases). 30% of infants born with congenital varicella syndrome die in the first month of life (Table 11).

Transmission

Person to person by direct contact, inhalation of aerosols from vesicular fluid of skin lesions of acute varicella and/or zoster, or aerosolized respiratory tract secretions.

Table 11 TIMING OF MATERNAL VARICELLA INFECTION AND POTENTIAL OUTCOME IN FETUS

Period of Gestation of Infected Mother	Potential Outcome in the Fetus
7 to 28 weeks	Fetal varicella syndrome
1 to 28 weeks	Neonatal/childhood herpes zoster
2 weeks before delivery	Neonatal chickenpox
*5 days before or after delivery	Neonatal disseminated chickenpox with septicemia and increased mortality of up to 30%

*potentially the most severe outcome for the fetus

Incubation period

Incubation period is 14 to 16 days after exposure to rash. The maximal period of contagiousness is 1 to 2 days before onset of the rash until all the lesions have crusted. In cases where there is only a maculopapular rash, person is contagious until the rash disappears.

Prevention

Post-exposure
   a. Varicella Zoster Immune Globulin (VariZIG) administered intramuscularly from 96 hours to 10 days after exposure. Recommended dose is based upon kg of body weight: 62.5 units (0.5 vial) for children weighing ≤2.0 kg; 125 units (1 vial) for children weighing 2.1 to 10 kg; 250 units (2 vials) for children weighing 10.1 to 20 kg; 375 units

(3 vials) for children weighing 20.1 to 30 kg; 500 units (4 vials) for children weighing 30.1 to 40 kg; and 625 units (5 vials) for all people weighing >40 kg. If VariZIG not available, IVIG given intravenously may be used at a dose of 400 mg/kg.

b. Prophylactic administration of oral acyclovir beginning 7 days after exposure may also prevent or attenuate varicella disease in healthy children. There is no information on whether prophylactic oral acyclovir is protective for adults or immunocompromised people. Prophylactic dosing of acyclovir is 20 mg/kg per dose, administered 4 times per day with a maximum daily dose of 3200 mg or valacyclovir 20 mg/kg per dose, administered 3 times per day with a maximum daily dose of 3000 mg. This should be continued for 7 days.

c. Varicella vaccine administered ideally within 3 days but up to 5 days after exposure (followed by a second dose of vaccine at least 28 days after the first dose in persons 13 years of age and older) may prevent or modify disease.

d. Because vaccine is contraindicated in pregnancy, a pregnant woman with no evidence of immunity (either prior infection or vaccine) with significant varicella exposure is a candidate for acyclovir prophylactic therapy.

Preexposure

a. Varicella vaccine is a live, attenuated viral vaccine that is given subcutaneously as a 2 dose series. For persons 13 years of age and older, the second dose should be given at least 28 days after first dose. The vaccine should be stored in a frost-free freezer at an average temperature of $-15°C$ ($+5°F$) or colder.

Effectiveness

Effectiveness is 86% against varicella infection and 95% against severe disease after one dose, and 98% after 2 doses.

Duration of protection

Appears to be long lasting after two doses (at least 25 years).

Precautions and contraindications to varicella vaccine

Contraindications

1. History of a serious reaction (e.g., anaphylaxis) after a previous dose of varicella vaccine or to a varicella vaccine component.
2. Pregnancy currently or in a patient that may become pregnant within 1 month.
3. Any malignant condition, including blood dyscrasia, leukemia, lymphoma, or any type, or other malignant neoplasm affecting the bone marrow or lymphatic system.
4. A patient receiving high-dose systemic immunosuppression therapy (e.g., two weeks or more of daily prednisone or equivalent of 20 mg or more [or 2 mg/kg or more for body weight]).
5. Family history of congenital or hereditary immunodeficiency in a first-degree relative (e.g., parents, siblings) when the immunocompetence of the potential vaccine recipient has not been clinically substantiated or verified by a laboratory.
6. A child age 1 year or older with CD4+ T-lymphocyte percentages less than 15% or a child, adolescent, or adult age

6 years or older with CD4+ T-lymphocyte count less than 200 cells per microliter.

7. For combination MMRV only (approved only for use in children 1 through 12 years of age), primary or acquired immunodeficiency, including immunosuppression associated with AIDS or other clinical manifestations of HIV infections, cellular immunodeficiency, hypogammaglobulinemia, and dysgammaglobulinemia.

Precautions

1. Receipt within the previous 11 months of antibody-containing blood products (specific interval depends on product).
2. Moderate to severe acute illness with or without fever.

Frequently asked questions

Can an infant younger than 12 months of age receive the varicella vaccine if they were exposed to the chickenpox or zoster virus?

The **minimum age** for varicella vaccine is 12 months. Vaccination is *not* recommended for infants younger than 12 months of age even as post-exposure prophylaxis. A healthy infant should receive no specific treatment or vaccination after exposure to VZV.

Should a dose of varicella vaccine be given to infants younger than 12 months of age if they are traveling internationally?

Varicella vaccine is neither approved nor recommended for children younger than 12 months of age in any situation.

If a child inadvertently receives zoster vaccine instead of varicella vaccine, does that vaccine dose count?
The administration of zoster vaccine instead of varicella vaccine is a serious vaccine administration error and procedures, and safeguards should be put in place to prevent this error from happening again. The dose of zoster vaccine can be counted as one dose of varicella vaccine, and if the error occurred for the first dose, the person should receive the second dose of varicella vaccine on schedule.

Should a child who had chickenpox prior to their first birthday get the first dose of varicella vaccine at age 1 year?
If the child had confirmed varicella disease or laboratory evidence of prior disease, it is not necessary to vaccinate regardless of age at infection. If there is any question that the illness was actually varicella, the child should be vaccinated.

Is it recommended that children who received one varicella dose 12 years ago at age 1 year, be vaccinated with a second dose at this time?
Yes. The current CDC recommendation is for two doses of the varicella vaccine regardless of age, for anyone school age and older without evidence of immunity. For everyone whose varicella immunity is based on vaccination, 2 doses of varicella vaccine are recommended.

If a child or adult has not had documented chickenpox but has had shingles, is varicella vaccination still recommended?
No. Shingles is caused by varicella zoster virus, the same virus that causes chickenpox. A history of shingles based on a health-care provider diagnosis is evidence of immunity to

chickenpox. A person who has had shingles does not need to be vaccinated against varicella.

If a patient has a very mild case of chickenpox (less than 10 lesions), are they considered immune or should they receive the varicella vaccine?
A case of chickenpox, whether it is mild, moderate or severe, produces immunity to varicella. A patient with a reliable history of chickenpox does not need to receive the varicella vaccine. However, if there is any doubt about the diagnosis, it is best to vaccinate the patient. There is no harm in vaccinating a patient who may already be immune.

Should an infant receive the varicella vaccine if they are living in a household with a person who is pregnant or someone who is immunocompromised?
Yes. Based on available data, healthy children are unlikely to transmit the vaccine virus and transmission of vaccine virus to household contacts has rarely been documented. Transmission of the vaccine virus occurs almost exclusively when the vaccinated person develops a rash following vaccination.

What are the recommendations for the use of varicella vaccine in children with HIV or other immunodeficiencies?
The CDC recommends the use of varicella vaccine in children with humoral but not cellular immunodeficiencies. Single antigen varicella vaccine should be considered for HIV-infected children age 1 through 8 years with CD4+ T-lymphocyte percentages greater than or equal to 15% or for children age 9 years and older with CD4+ T-lymphocyte counts greater

than or equal to 200 cells per microliter. Eligible children should receive two doses of varicella vaccine with a 3-month interval between doses.

Should healthcare personnel avoid contact with immunocompromised patients after receiving varicella vaccine?
No. This is not necessary unless the person who was vaccinated develops a rash. If the vaccinated person develops a rash 7 to 21 days following vaccination, they should avoid prolonged close contact with a pregnant or immunosuppressed household contact or patient that is known to be susceptible to varicella, until the rash resolves.

What should be done in the situation in which hospital employees claim that they have had chickenpox; however, their varicella antibody titers show no antibodies?
If the health-care employee's history of chickenpox cannot be verified, the employee should receive two doses of varicella vaccine at least 4 weeks apart.

A health professions student (e.g., medical, nursing, dental, physical therapy, etc.) received 2 valid, appropriately spaced, documented doses of varicella vaccine. Subsequently a titer was drawn for whatever reason and the titer was negative. Is it recommended to revaccinate this individual with 2 doses of varicella vaccine?
No. Documented receipt of two doses of varicella vaccine supersedes results of subsequent serologic testing. Most commercially available tests for varicella antibody are not sensitive enough to detect vaccine-induced antibody, which

is why it is *not* recommended to perform post-vaccination testing.

Is receipt of a single documented dose of zoster vaccine proof of varicella immunity in a health-care employee who has no other evidence of immunity?

No. Receipt of zoster vaccine is not proof of prior varicella disease. Per the CDC, acceptable evidence of varicella immunity in healthcare personnel includes: (1) documentation of two doses of varicella vaccine given at least 28 days apart, (2) history of varicella or herpes zoster based on physician diagnosis, (3) laboratory evidence of immunity, or (4) laboratory confirmation of disease. If a health-care employee has already received a dose of zoster vaccine but has no evidence of immunity to varicella, the zoster dose can be considered the first dose of the two dose varicella vaccine series.

How soon after varicella exposure does the varicella vaccine need to be administered if it is used in a postexposure setting?

Varicella vaccine is effective in preventing chickenpox or reducing the severity of the disease if used within 72 hours (3 days), and possibly up to 5 days, after exposure. Not every exposure to varicella leads to infection, so for future immunity, varicella vaccine should be given, even if more than 5 days have passed since the exposure.

What are the circumstances in which a varicella titer should be obtained after vaccination?

Obtaining postvaccination serologic testing is *not* recommended in any group, including healthcare personnel.

Should all pregnant women have serology screening for varicella?

No. Serologic testing for varicella should only be considered for women who do not have evidence of immunity (either a reliable history or chickenpox or documented vaccination). Once a person has been found to be seropositive, it is not necessary to test them again in the future.

What should be done in the situation where a full-term, healthy, 2-month-old infant was exposed to their mother and another household contact with varicella for the last week?

There is no evidence that healthy full-term infants born to women in whom varicella occurs more than 48 hours after delivery are at increased risk for serious complications from the disease. Varicella zoster immune globulin (VariZIG) can be given up to 10 days after exposure, but it is only recommended for newborn infants whose mothers have signs and symptoms of varicella around the time of delivery (5 days before to 2 days after), hospitalized premature infants born at 28 or more weeks gestation whose mothers do not have evidence of immunity to varicella, or hospitalized premature infants born at less than 28 weeks of gestation or who weigh 1,000 grams or less at birth regardless of their mothers' evidence of immunity to varicella. In the above situation, VariZIG would not be recommended. If the infant develops varicella, it would be managed as it would be for any healthy child.

HERPES ZOSTER (SHINGLES)

Did you know that:

- The term *herpes zoster* is derived from the Greek word *herpes* meaning creeping and *zoster* meaning a beltlike

binding or girdle and describes a herpes zoster rash encir-
cling the waist.

- Otto von Bismarck ("Iron Chancellor" and architect of the
unification of Germany), James H. Doolittle (American
aviation pioneer), Golda Meir (fourth prime minister of
Israel), and Charles Lindbergh ("Lucky Lindy," aviator and
explorer) all suffered from severe bouts of herpes zoster
(shingles).

Herpes zoster is caused by the reactivation of the varicella
zoster (chickenpox) virus and may occur years or decades after
primary illness with chickenpox. It is generally associated with
normal aging and with anything that causes reduced immunocompetence (e.g., bone marrow and solid organ transplants,
hematologic malignancies and solid tumors, HIV, immunosuppressive medications). Other risk factors include: female gender, white race, trauma, surgery and persons with early varicella
(e.g., varicella in utero or early infancy). One in three persons
will develop herpes zoster sometime during their lifetime with
an estimated 1 million cases occurring annually in the United
States.

Clinical features include a prodromal illness of headache,
photophobia, malaise, fever, and abnormal skin sensation or
pain in the affected area. This is followed by the development
of the zoster rash that is unilateral involving 1 to 3 adjacent
dermatomes. Thoracic, cervical, and ophthalmic areas are most
commonly involved. The rash initially starts as erythematous and maculopapular and then evolves into vesicles over
several days before crusting. Full resolution of the rash may
take 2 to 4 weeks. Occasionally the rash does not develop but
patient continues with abnormal skin sensation and pain in the
affected area.

Complications of herpes zoster include:

a. Postherpetic neuralgia, the most common complication, develops in 10% to 34% of people. It ranges from mild-to-excruciating constant or intermittent pain occurring after the resolution of the rash. The pain may persist for weeks, months, or even years and may be completely debilitating. Risk factors include age ≥50 years and severe zoster disease.

b. Herpes zoster ophthalmicus occurs in up to 15% of cases and can lead to reduced vision and even blindness. If untreated, 50% to 70% develop acute ocular complications.

c. Secondary infection of the herpes zoster rash, which may lead to permanent scarring or changes in skin pigmentation.

d. Neurologic complications including encephalitis, ventriculitis, cranial nerve palsies, meningoencephalitis, myelitis and ischemic stroke syndrome.

e. Rarely varicella zoster virus viremia can lead to pneumonia, hepatitis, DIC.

Transmission

Transmission is person to person via direct contact with zoster lesions, however, airborne transmission may occur in certain settings. A person is contagious from the time the rash erupts until the lesions are crusted. Transmission may be decreased by covering the lesions and preventing contact.

Prevention

a. Herpes Zoster Vaccine which is a live, attenuated varicella vaccine that contains 14 times the amount of virus compared to regular varicella vaccine. It is administered subcutaneously as a single dose and must be **stored in a freezer** at all times. It is recommended for all adults ≥60 years of age **whether or not** they have reported a prior episode of shingles. Persons with chronic medical conditions may be vaccinated unless a contraindication or precaution exists. Contraindications for vaccination include severe allergic reaction after exposure to any component of the vaccine, primary or acquired immunodeficiency and immunosuppressive therapy.

Contraindications and Precautions with Herpes zoster vaccine

Contraindications

1. Severe allergic reaction (e.g., anaphylaxis) after a previous dose or to a vaccine component.
2. Known severe immunodeficiency (e.g., hematologic and solid tumors, receipt of chemotherapy, or long-term immunosuppressive therapy, patients with HIV who are severely immunocompromised).
3. Pregnancy. Women should not become pregnant for at least 4 weeks after receiving the zoster vaccine.

Precautions

1. Moderate or severe acute illness with or without fever.
2. Receipt of specific antiviral agents (e.g., acyclovir, famciclovir, or valacyclovir) 24 hours before vaccination. The use of these antiviral agents should be avoided for 14 days after receiving the vaccine as it will reduce the immune response to the vaccine.

Effectiveness

Reduces risk for developing zoster by 51%, post-herpetic neuralgia by 66.5% and overall severity and duration of disease by 61%.

Duration of protection

Unknown. No booster dose of vaccine is recommended at this time.

Frequently asked questions

Zoster vaccine is approved by the FDA for people age 50 years and older. Does the CDC recommend that health-care providers vaccinate people in their 50s?
CDC does not currently recommend the use of zoster vaccine in people 50 to 59 years of age. The reasons for not vaccinating this population include: (1) even though the burden of herpes zoster disease increases after age 50, disease rates are lower in this age group than they are in persons 60 years of age and older; (2) there is insufficient evidence for long-term protection provided by the vaccine; and (3) persons vaccinated at younger than age 60 years may not be protected when the incidence of zoster and its complication are highest. Zoster vaccine is approved by the FDA for persons aged 50 through 59 years and health-care providers may choose to vaccinate persons in this age group despite the absence of a CDC recommendation.

Is there an upper age limit for receipt of the zoster vaccine?
There is no upper age limit for zoster vaccine. The incidence of herpes zoster increases with increasing age; an estimated 50%

of persons living until age 85 years will develop zoster. CDC recommends the vaccine for everyone age 60 years and older, even though vaccine efficacy decreases with an increase in the age of the vaccine recipient. With increasing age at vaccination, the vaccine is more effective in reducing the severity of zoster and post-herpetic neuralgia than in reducing the occurrence of disease.

Is it necessary to ask when a person has ever had chickenpox or shingles prior to administering zoster vaccine?
No. All persons aged 60 years of age and older, whether or not they have a history of chickenpox or shingles, should receive zoster vaccine unless they have a medical contraindication to vaccination. Serologic studies show that almost everyone born in the United States before 1980 has had chickenpox. It is also not recommended or necessary to test for varicella antibody prior to administering the vaccine.

How soon after a case of shingles can a person receive the zoster vaccine?
The general rule for any vaccine is to wait until the patient is over the acute stage of the illness and symptoms have resolved. A recent case of shingles is expected to boost the immunity of the person to varicella and administering zoster vaccine to a person whose immunity was recently boosted by a case of shingles might reduce the effectiveness of the vaccine. CDC does not have specific recommendations for this issue, however, it may be wise to defer zoster vaccination for 6 to 12 months after the shingles has resolved so that the vaccine can produce a more effective boost to immunity.

What should be done in the situation where a child received zoster vaccine instead of varicella vaccine?

This is a serious vaccine administration error and the event needs to be documented and procedures put in place to prevent this from occurring again. Zoster vaccine contains 14 times as much varicella vaccine virus as varicella vaccine; however, no specific action needs to be taken in response to this error. If this was the child's first dose of varicella-containing vaccine, they will still need the second dose of varicella-containing vaccine given as per the recommended schedule.

What should be done in the situation where a 60-year-old patient was inadvertently given varicella vaccine instead of zoster vaccine?

If a provider inadvertently administers varicella vaccine to a person for whom zoster vaccine is indicated, the dose should not be considered valid and the patient should be administered a dose of zoster vaccine during the same visit. If the error is not immediately detected, a dose of zoster vaccine should be administered 4 weeks after the varicella vaccine dose to prevent potential blunting of the immune response to 2 doses of live, attenuated viral vaccine.

If a 65-year-old patient has an underlying condition that requires monthly treatment with intravenous immune globulin (IVIG), can they receive the zoster vaccine?

Yes. The concern about interference by circulating antibody in the IVIG, applies to varicella and MMR vaccines but not to zoster vaccine. The amount of antigen in zoster vaccine is so substantial that it offsets any effect of any circulating herpes zoster antibody that may be in the IVIG.

When can a patient who is receiving immunosuppressive chemotherapy receive zoster vaccine?

If a patient is receiving or has recently received cancer chemotherapy, it is recommended to wait 3 months after the therapy is discontinued before administering zoster vaccine. If the patient was receiving high-dose steroids, isoantibodies, immune mediators, or immunomodulators, it is recommended to wait 1 month after the therapy is discontinued before administering zoster vaccine. If the person was receiving low doses of methotrexate, azathioprine, or 6-mercaptopurine, it is not necessary to wait as these therapies are not considered immunosuppressive.

Is there any reason to delay administration of zoster vaccination in a healthy person 60 years of age and older who has frequent contact with an unvaccinated infant or an immunocompromised person?

Neither one of these situation is a reason to delay administration of zoster vaccine. There are no special contact precautions that are needed if a person who receives zoster vaccine has close household or occupational contact with persons who are at risk for developing severe varicella or zoster infection. The only exception is in the rare instance when a person develops a varicella-like rash after receiving zoster vaccine. If a rash develops, the vaccinated person should restrict contact with an immunocompromised person if the immunocompromised person is susceptible to varicella.

PNEUMOCOCCAL DISEASE

Did you know that:

- Charles Bronson, actor; James Brown, the "Godfather of Soul"; Leo Tolstoy, author of *War and Peace*; Rene Descartes, French philosopher, mathematician, and scientist; and horror film actor Boris Karloff all died from pneumococcal pneumonia.
- The organism, *Streptococcus pneumoniae*, was first identified concurrently in 1881 in France by Louis Pasteur and in the United States by George Sternberg.
- Adults 65 years and older comprise about 15% of the population of the United States but account for one third of all the cases of invasive pneumococcal disease.
- In 1911, Sir Almroth Wright, a scientist renowned for his work developing an effective vaccine for typhoid fever, was sent to South Africa to develop and test a pneumococcal vaccine in order to alleviate the burden of epidemic disease in gold miners. Despite vaccinating over 50,000 miners and claiming his results showed that the vaccine worked, his data did not hold up well to scrutiny. This left him with the unfortunate nickname "Sir Almost Right."

Capsular polysaccharides are an important determinant of pathogenicity and form the basis for classifying pneumococci by serotypes. Ninety-four different serotypes have been identified to date.

Since the introduction of routine infant PCV-7 vaccine in 2000, indirect vaccine effects have reduced invasive pneumococcal infections among unvaccinated persons of all ages, including those aged ≥65 years. Among persons 18 to 49 years, 50 to 64 years, and ≥65 years, rates of IPD decreased 40%, 18%, and 37%, respectively. However, IPD remains an important cause of illness and death with an estimated 43,500 cases and 5,000 deaths occurring among persons of all ages; 36,540 cases of IPD (e.g., pneumonia, bacteremia, meningitis) and 4,900 deaths (98%) are seen in persons >50 years of age. The highest mortality rates are seen among the elderly (17.4% for those ≥65 years of age and 20.6% for those >80 years of age) with persons ≥65 years of age accounting for more than 50% of all deaths from IPD.

The conjugate pneumococcal vaccine has had a major impact on the incidence of invasive disease among young children, resulting in a 99% decrease in disease caused by the seven serotypes in PCV7 and serotype 6A, a serotype against which PCV7 provides some cross-protection. These decreases have been offset partially by increases in invasive disease caused by serotypes not included in PCV7. Indirect effects of the conjugate vaccine have reduced invasive pneumococcal infections among unvaccinated persons of all ages. However, pneumococcal pneumonia and IPD remain important causes of illness and death with an estimated 400,000 hospitalizations annually for pneumococcal pneumonia; 12,000 cases of bacteremia with a case-fatality rate of 20% (and up to 60% in the elderly); and 3,000-6,000 cases of meningitis with a case-fatality rate of 22% in adults and 8% in children.

Transmission

Person to person by respiratory droplet contact. Viral upper respiratory infections, including influenza, can predispose to pneumococcal infection and transmission.

Incubation period

Varies by type of infection but can be as short as 1 to 3 days.

Persons at Increased Risk for Pneumococcal Disease

Individuals at increased risk for pneumococcal disease include: those with chronic heart disease (especially those with cyanotic heart disease and cardiac failure), chronic lung disease (including asthma especially if treated with prolonged high-dose oral steroids), diabetes mellitus, cerebrospinal fluid leaks, cochlear implant, sickle cell disease and other hemoglobinopathies, chronic or acquired asplenia or splenic dysfunction, HIV infection, diseases associated with treatment with immunosuppressive drugs or radiation therapy (e.g., malignant neoplasms, leukemias, lymphomas, and Hodgkin disease, or solid organ transplantation), congenital immunodeficiency (e.g. B and T lymphocyte deficiency, complement deficiencies [especially C1, C2, C3, and C4 deficiency], phagocyte disorders, alcoholism, chronic liver disease, cigarette smokers).

Prevention

Pneumococcal vaccine—2 types of pneumococcal vaccine available

a. 23-valent polysaccharide vaccine (PPSV23)
b. 13-valent protein conjugate vaccine (PCV13)—each capsular polysaccharide is individually conjugated to a nontoxic variant of diphtheria toxin carrier protein, CRM_{197}.

PPSV23 contains 23 pneumococcal serotypes that account for 85% to 90% of invasive disease in persons >2 years of age. PPSV23 is effective in preventing bacteremia, bacteremic pneumonia, and meningitis with an efficacy of 56% to 81%. The vaccine does not prevent non-bacteremic pneumonia.

PCV13 contains 13 pneumococcal serotypes that account for 92% of invasive disease. PCV13 has been proven effective in preventing bacteremia, pneumonia (with and without bacteremia), meningitis, otitis media with an efficacy of 90% to 100% against the various pneumococcal serotypes contained in the vaccine. This is a routinely recommended vaccine of childhood given as a 4 dose series at 2, 4, 6, and 15 to 18 months. Doses routinely may be given up to 5 years of age. Persons between 6 and 18 years of age who are at increased risk for IPD because of functional or anatomic asplenia, sickle cell disease, HIV or other immunocompromising conditions, cochlear implant, or CSF leak should receive a single dose of PCV13 regardless of whether they have received PPSV23 or PCV7 in the past. Conjugate vaccines like PCV13 also decrease nasopharyngeal colonization and indirectly reduce the risk of invasive pneumococcal disease in unvaccinated contacts.

The CDC has expanded recommendations for use of PCV13 vaccine in adults 19 years and older with certain immunocompromising conditions. In these situations vaccine is given as a single dose.

The CDC recommends *both* PCV13 and PPSV23 for

- All adults age 65 years and older
- Adults age 19 to 64 years with:
  - Conditions or treatments that affect the immune system (such as: HIV, lymphoma, leukemia, or Hodgkin

disease, chronic kidney disease, radiation therapy, or certain long-term corticosteroid use, multiple myeloma

- Functional or anatomic asplenia
- Cochlear implants or cerebrospinal fluid (CSF) leaks
- Organ transplant
- Congenital or acquired immune deficiencies

If a patient has received at least one dose of PPSV23, a single dose of PCV13 is recommended at least 1 year after the last PPSV23 dose. If needed, a second PPSV23 dose is recommended for immunosuppressed and asplenic persons at least 8 weeks after PCV13 and five years after the first PPSV23.

If the patient has not previously been immunized with PPSV23, a dose of PCV13 should be given followed 1 year later by a dose of PPSV23.

CDC recommends *only* PPSV23 for the following adults age 19 to 64 years:

- Those with chronic conditions such as asthma, diabetes, lung, heart, or liver disease, or alcoholism
- Cigarette smokers
- Residents of nursing homes or other long-term care facilities

These individuals should receive a dose of PCV13 when they reach age 65 years.

Vaccine efficacy

PPSV23 in older adults has an efficacy of about 75% against invasive pneumococcal disease. In the US, PCV13 in children ≤5 years of age has an effectiveness of 86% against IPD.

Contraindications and precautions for pneumococcal vaccines

Contraindications
1. For PCV13—Severe allergic reaction (e.g., anaphylaxis) after a previous dose or to a vaccine component, including to any vaccine containing diphtheria toxoid.
2. For PPSV23—Severe allergic reaction (e.g., anaphylaxis) after a previous dose or to a vaccine component.

Precautions
For both PCV13 and PPSV23—moderate or severe acute illness with or without fever

Frequently asked questions

What should be done in the situation where a 2-month-old was mistakenly given PPSV23 instead of PCV13?
PPSV23 is not effective in infants and children less than 24 months of age. PPSV23 given at this age should not be considered to be part of the pneumococcal vaccination series. PCV13 should be administered as soon as possible after the error was discovered.

Which children should receive PPSV23 vaccine (in addition to PCV13)? At what age should they receive PPSV23?
PPSV23 is recommended for children with an immunocompromising condition, functional or anatomic asplenia, and for immunocompetent children with chronic heart disease, chronic lung disease, diabetes mellitus, CSF leaks, or cochlear implants. One dose of PPSV23 should be administered to children age 2 years and older at least 8 weeks after the child has

received the final dose of PCV13. Children with an immuno-compromising condition, or functional or anatomic asplenia should receive a second dose of PPSV23 five years after the first PPSV23 dose.

Can PPSV23 be given to a pregnant woman with asthma?
Yes. PPSV23 is recommended in pregnancy if some other risk factor is present (e.g., on the basis of medical, occupational, lifestyle, or other indications).

Given that PPSV23 is indicated for smokers age 19 through 64 years, should adults who use smokeless tobacco products (e.g., chewing tobacco) also be vaccinated?
No. The CDC does not identify people who use smokeless tobacco products as being at increased risk for pneumococcal disease or as being in a risk group for vaccination.

Is PCV13 recommended for adults age 19 through 64 years who smoke?
No. PCV13 is only recommended for adults 19 through 64 years at increased risk for invasive pneumococcal disease because of an immunocompromising condition, asplenia, cerebrospinal fluid leak or cochlear implant.

Is obstructive sleep apnea (OSA) considered a chronic pulmonary disease which would require PPSV23 vaccination for adults under 65 years of age?
OSA alone is not an indication for vaccination with PPSV23 for persons 2 through 64 years of age. Persons with OSA often have other pulmonary conditions (e.g., chronic obstructive pulmonary disease) that would put them at increased risk

for invasive pneumococcal disease, for which they should be vaccinated.

Can PPSV23 and PCV13 be administered at the same office visit?
No. PCV13 and PPSV23 should not be given at the same visit. If PCV13 is indicated, administer it if at least 1 year has passed since the previous dose of PPSV23 or if no doses of PPSV23 have previously been received. Then wait at least 8 weeks for adults with immune compromise and at least 1 year for all other adults to administer PPSV23.

If an adult who is 19 through 64 years of age has already gotten one or more doses of PPSV23, when should they get PCV13, if indicated?
PCV13 should be administered at least 1 year after the previous dose of PPSV23 was administered. For those who require additional doses of PPSV23, the first such dose should be given at least 8 weeks after PCV13 and at least 5 years since the most recent dose of PPSV23.

If a patient has had laboratory confirmed pneumococcal pneumonia or other invasive pneumococcal disease, do they still need to be vaccinated with PCV13 and/or PPSV23?
Yes. There are more than 90 known serotypes of pneumococcus. PCV13 contains 13 serotypes and PPSV23 contains 23 different serotypes. Infection with one serotype does not necessarily produce immunity to other serotypes. Therefore, if a person is a candidate for vaccination, they should receive it even after one or more episodes of invasive pneumococcal disease.

Do patients who were vaccinated with one or two doses of PPSV23 before age 65 years need an additional dose of PPSV23 at age 65 or later?

Yes. Patients who received one or two doses of PPSV23 for any indication at age 64 years of younger should receive an additional dose of PPSV23 vaccine at age 65 years or older if at least 5 years have elapsed since their previous PPSV23 dose.

If an adult age 65 years or older has already received one dose of PCV13 before age 65 for an appropriate indication, should another dose of PCV13 be given at age 65?

No. If a dose of PCV13 was already received before age 65 for an appropriate indication, no additional PCV13 doses are needed. A dose of PPSV23 should be administered at age 65 and at least 1 year following the PCV13 dose.

If patient over 65 years of age and has recently received one dose of PPSV23 is diagnosed with a medical condition that places them at increased risk for pneumococcal disease and its complications, should a second dose of PPSV23 be given in 5 years because of the underlying medical condition?

No. Individuals who are first vaccinated with PPSV23 at age 65 years or older should receive only one dose, regardless of any underlying medical condition that they may have developed.

Should the dose of PCV13 be repeated if given less than 1 year after a dose of PPSV23? If yes, what is the interval between doses?

No, if inadvertently administered sooner than the recommended interval, no repeat dose is recommended. The two vaccines should never be given during the same visit.

If I inadvertently administer PPSV23 less than 8 weeks after PCV13, do I need to repeat the dose of either vaccine?

No. Administration of PPSV23 less than 8 weeks after PCV13 may increase risk for localized reaction at the injection site but remains a valid vaccination and should not be repeated; the PCV13 dose also remains valid and should not be repeated.

How many doses of PPSV23 can an adult get in a lifetime?

Some adults may be recommended to receive up to 3 doses of PPSV23 in a lifetime. Two doses of PPSV23, given 5 years apart, are indicated for adults with functional or anatomic asplenia and immunocompromising conditions before age 65 years. Those adults should then receive a third dose of PPSV23 at or after 65 years, as long as it's been at least 5 years since the previous dose.

How many doses of PCV13 can an adult get in a lifetime? Who/when?

All adults are recommended to receive 1 dose of PCV13 in a lifetime. If they received a dose of PCV13 prior to turning 65 years of age (due to a medical indication), they are not recommended an additional dose of PCV13 as part of the routine recommendation to administer PCV13 to all adults 65 years of age or older.

Can either PPSV23 and/or PCV13 be administered to patients with multiple sclerosis?

Yes. Multiple sclerosis is not a contraindication to any vaccine, including either of the pneumococcal vaccines.

When should patients (either children or adults) be vaccinated if they are scheduled to have either cochlear implant placement or an elective splenectomy?

It is preferable that the person planning to have the procedure have antibodies to pneumococcus at the time of the surgery. If possible, the appropriate vaccine should be administered prior to the cochlea implant or splenectomy. Infants and children 2 through 71 months of age should continue to receive PCV13 vaccine according to the recommended vaccine schedule.

MENINGOCOCCAL DISEASE

Did you know that:

- The "meningitis belt" refers to a region stretching across sub-Saharan Africa, which has seen recurring epidemics of meningococcal meningitis. An estimated 250,000 people developed meningitis and 25,000 died when the largest epidemic in recorded history spread through the region in 1996 and 1997. The Meningitis Vaccine Project has provided widespread vaccination with a low-cost conjugate meningococcal type A vaccine resulting in an 89% decrease in disease and an 83% decrease in deaths from 2009 to 2013.
- In the pre-antibiotic era, the case fatality rate from meningococcal disease was 70% to 85%. Today, despite effective antimicrobial therapy and state-of-the-art intensive care, the overall case fatality rate remains 10% to 15%.
- Many patients with severe meningococcal sepsis respond poorly to treatment with antimicrobial agents, steroids, or vasopressor agents, and death may occur within hours of onset.

Meningococcal disease is caused by the organism *Neisseria meningitidis* (encapsulated gram-negative diplococcus), which is strictly a human pathogen. Asymptomatic carriage is common with 10% of the general population and 25% to 30% of the adolescent/young adult population being carriers. Less than 1% of carriers will become symptomatic with disease. Most common clinical presentations of disease are meningitis accounting for about 50% of the cases with a 3% to 10% fatality rate and meningococcal sepsis (meningococcemia) accounting for 10% to 40% of cases with up to a 40% fatality rate. Both presentations may be associated with serious permanent sequelae. Fatality rates and rates of serious outcomes are significantly higher in the adolescent and young adult populations compared to general population (23% vs. 13%). Other clinical presentations that are less common include pneumonia, occult bacteremia, septic arthritis and otitis media.

Onset of disease can be nonspecific but often is abrupt and may progress rapidly over several hours. Patients develop fever, chills, sore throat, nausea and/or vomiting, general aches, diarrhea, headache, malaise, limb pain, abnormal skin color, cold hands and feet, and a rash that initially can be macular, maculopapular, petechial, or purpuric. In fulminant cases, purpura, limb ischemia, coagulopathy, pulmonary edema, shock with poor peripheral perfusion, hypotension, confusion, tachycardia, tachypnea and oliguria, coma, and death may occur in hours despite appropriate therapy. The signs and symptoms of meningococcal meningitis are indistinguishable from other causes of meningitis.

Complications and sequelae

a. Meningococcemia includes: skin scars from necrosis, limb loss from gangrene, renal insufficiency, septic arthritis, pneumonia, epiglottis, pericarditis

b. Meningitis includes: hearing loss, seizures, hemiparesis, spastic quadriplegia, cerebral infarction, cranial nerve palsies, cortical venous thrombophlebitis, mental retardation

Risk factors for disease include: impaired immunity (e.g., terminal complement component deficiency, properidin deficiency), functional or anatomic asplenia, nasopharyngeal irritation and disruption of the mucous membranes, social behaviors that predispose to exposure to secretions. Also persons traveling to or residing in countries where *N. meningitidis* is endemic; military recruits; persons attending summer camps and colleges who will be living in dormitory setting; microbiologists, laboratory personnel, and other healthcare workers who are routinely exposed to *N. meningitidis*.

Most common serogroups causing disease include: serogroup A, serogroup B, serogroup C, serogroup Y, serogroup X, and serogroup W-135. Serogroup distribution varies over time and geographically. Most common serogroups in US are B, C, Y, and W135; in Europe serogroup B, in African meningitis belt serogroup A, in Saudi Arabia serogroup W-135 and in New Zealand serogroup B.

Transmission

Person to person through contact with droplets from the respiratory tract. Transmission requires close contact. Close contact defined as:

a. Household contact, especially children younger than 2 years of age
b. Child-care or preschool contact at any time during 7 days before onset of illness
c. Direct exposure to index patient's secretions through kissing or through sharing toothbrushes or eating utensils,

markers of close social contact, at any time during 7 days before onset of illness

d. Mouth-to-mouth resuscitation, unprotected contact during endotracheal intubation at any time 7 days before onset of illness

e. Frequently sleeping in same dwelling as index patient during 7 days before onset of illness

f. Passengers seated directly next to the index case during airline flights lasting more than 8 hours

Incubation period

Incubation period is 1 to 10 days but usually less than 4 days.

Prevention

Postexposure

a. Antibiotic chemoprophylaxis—**regardless of immunization status**, close contacts of all persons with invasive meningococcal disease are at high risk and should receive post-exposure chemoprophylaxis (Table 12). Chemoprophylaxis ideally should be initiated within 24 hours after the index patient is diagnosed; prophylaxis given more than 2 weeks after exposure has little value.

b. Quadrivalent meningococcal conjugate vaccine (MenACWY) should be given **in addition** to antibiotic chemoprophylaxis to those persons who have not previously been immunized. Vaccine is given intramuscularly.

Preexposure

Table 15 shows the available meningococcal vaccines against meningococcal serotypes A, C, W, Y.

a. Quadrivalent meningococcal conjugate vaccine (MenACWY)—routinely recommended vaccination for

Table 12 ANTIBIOTIC CHEMOPROPHYLAXIS AGENTS FOR CLOSE CONTACTS OF PATIENTS WITH INVASIVE MENINGOCOCCAL DISEASE

Antibiotic	Dose	Duration	Cautions
Rifampin	10 mg/kg PO q 12 hours (max 600 mg)	2 days	Can interfere with efficacy of oral contraceptives and some seizure and anticoagulant medications. Not recommended to be used in pregnant women
Ceftriaxone			
<15 years of age	125 mg IM	Single dose	
≥15 years of age	250 mg IM	Single dose	
Ciprofloxacin	20 mg/kg PO (max 500 mg)	Single dose	Not recommended to be used in pregnant women
Azithromycin	10 mg/kg PO (max 500 mg)	Single dose	Not routinely recommended

all adolescents 11 to 18 years of age (Table 13), persons with HIV ≥2 months of age, and persons 2 to 54 years of age with persistent complement component deficiency or functional or anatomic asplenia. Vaccine should also be given to other persons at increased risk for meningococcal disease (see above risk factors for disease).

All persons ≥2 months of age with HIV should routinely receive meningococcal vaccine. The number of doses and dosing schedule are shown in the Table 14.

Routine 2-dose primary series administered 2 months apart for: persons 2 to 54 years of age with persistent complement

Table 13 SCHEDULE FOR ROUTINE DOSING OF ADOLESCENTS

Initial (primary) dose	Booster dose
11–12 years (preferred timing)	16 years
13–15 years	16–18 years
≥ 16 years	No booster needed

component deficiency, functional or anatomic asplenia and adolescents with HIV infection.

A dose should be given to persons traveling to or residing in countries where *N. meningitidis* is endemic; military recruits;

Table 14 MENINGOCOCCAL VACCINE SCHEDULE IN PATIENTS WITH HIV

Primary vaccination	
<2 years	4 doses of Menveo (MenACWY-CRM) at 2,4,6 and 12–15 months
	2 doses of Menatra (MenACWY) at 9–23 months, 12 weeks apart
≥2 years	2 doses of Menveo or Menactra, 8 to 12 weeks apart
Booster dose	
<7 years at previous dose	Additional dose of Menveo or Menactra 3 years after primary series; boosters should be repeated every 5 years thereafter
≥7 years at previous dose	Additional dose of Menveo or Menactra 5 years after primary series; boosters should be repeated every 5 years thereafter

Table 15 CURRENTLY AVAILABLE MENINGOCOCCAL VACCINES

	Trade Name	Type of Vaccine	Meningococcal Serogroups covered
MPSV4	Menomune®	Polysaccharide	A, C, W, Y
MenACWY	Menactra®	Conjugate	A, C, W, Y
MenACWY-CRM	Menveo®	Conjugate	A, C, W, Y
Hib-MenCY-TT	MenHibrix®	Conjugate	C, Y (and *Haemophilus influenzae* type b [Hib])

persons attending summer camps and colleges who will be living in dormitory setting; microbiologists, laboratory personnel, and other health-care workers who are routinely exposed to *N. meningitidis*. Booster dose may be given 5 years after initial dose if the person continues to be in a situation of increased risk.

Vaccination with a meningococcal conjugate vaccine is recommended for infants aged 2 through 23 months at increased risk for meningococcal disease. Infants at increased risk for meningococcal disease are:

- those with persistent complement component deficiencies (C3, C5–C9, properdin, factor D, and factor H),
- those with functional or anatomic asplenia (including sickle cell disease),
- healthy infants in communities with a meningococcal disease outbreak for which vaccination is recommended, and
- those traveling to or residing in areas where meningococcal disease is hyperendemic or epidemic.

b. Meningococcal serogroup B vaccine (MenB)—currently has a category B recommendation which means that the MenB vaccine series may be administered to adolescents and young adults aged 16 to 23 years to provide short term protection against most strains of serogroup B meningococcal disease based on the clinical judgment of the health-care provider for the individual patient (weighing the risk and benefits). The preferred age for MenB vaccination is 16 to 18 years.

There are two MenB vaccines that are licensed in the U.S. MenB vaccine should either be administered as a 2-dose or a 3-dose series of MenB-FHbp (Trumenba) or a 2-dose series of MenB-4C (Bexsero). The two MenB vaccines are not interchangeable; the same vaccine product must be used for all doses. Both vaccines may be administered concomitantly with other vaccines indicated for this age group.

MenB-FHbp (Trumenba)—2 dose series at 0 and 6 months
    3 dose series given at 0, 1 2, and 6 months.
MenB-4C (Bexsero)—2-dose series given at least 1 month apart.

Efficacy

MenACYW—80% to 100% for the serotypes contained in the vaccine.

Duration of immunity

For MCV4 vaccines, probably 3 years. Duration of immunity for MenB vaccines unknown.

Contraindications and precautions for meningococcal vaccines

Contraindications

Severe allergic reaction (e.g., anaphylaxis) after a previous dose or to a vaccine component.

Precautions

Moderate or severe acute illness with or without fever

Frequently asked questions

Is meningococcal polysaccharide vaccine appropriate for adolescents?

Only the quadrivalent meningococcal conjugate vaccine (MCV4) is recommended for adolescents. However, an initial dose of meningococcal vaccine administered as polysaccharide vaccine can be counted as valid. The booster dose of meningococcal vaccine should always be quadrivalent meningococcal conjugate vaccine. If polysaccharide vaccine is inadvertently administered as the booster dose, revaccination with conjugate vaccine is recommended 8 weeks later.

Who is recommended to be vaccinated against meningococcal disease?

MCV4 is recommended for:

- All children and teens, aged 11 through 18 years of age
- People younger than 22 years of age if they are or will be a first-year college student living in a residential hall
- People aged 2 months and older with functional or anatomic asplenia (MenHibrix may be used for children age 6 weeks through 18 months in this group—vaccine only contains meningococcal serogroups C and Y)

- People aged 2 months and older who reside in or travel to certain countries in sub-Saharan Africa as well as to other countries for which meningococcal vaccine is recommended (e.g., travel to Mecca, Saudi Arabia, for the annual Hajj)
- Microbiologists who work with meningococcus bacteria in the laboratory

MenB is recommended for:

- People 10 years of age and older who have functional or anatomic asplenia
- People 10 years of age and older who have persistent complement component deficiency, or are at risk during an outbreak caused by a vaccine serogroup
- Microbiologists who work with meningococcus bacteria in the laboratory

Can adolescents receive quadrivalent meningococcal vaccine and serogroup B meningococcal vaccine at the same time?

Yes. Meningococcal and other vaccines may be administered during the same visit but at a different anatomic site if feasible.

Is meningococcal vaccination recommended for adolescents during outbreaks?

Yes. If a meningococcal disease outbreak is serogroup A, C, W, or Y, vaccination with quadrivalent meningococcal vaccine is recommended for adolescents identified as being at increased risk. If the meningococcal disease outbreak is serogroup B, adolescents identified as being at increased risk because of the outbreak should be vaccinated with serogroup B meningococcal vaccine.

Why isn't it recommended to administer the serogroup B meningococcal vaccine to all adolescents?

Administration of the serogroup B meningococcal vaccine to patients 16 through 23 years of age is left to the discretion of the clinician. Detailed efficacy and safety data for making policy recommendations are not yet available because these vaccines were licensed for use in the United States under an accelerated approval process. And the current burden of disease with this serotype is low. In the setting of an outbreak of serogroup B disease, vaccination would be appropriate.

How many doses of serogroup B meningococcal vaccine are necessary?

Both serogroup B meningococcal vaccines require more than one dose for maximum protection: two doses for Bexsero (0, ≥1 month after first dose) and two or three doses for Trumenba (0, 6 months after 1st dose or 0, 1–2 after 1st dose and 6 months after 1st dose). The same vaccine product must be used for all doses.

Are there any groups for whom a booster dose of MenB vaccine is recommended after completion of the primary series?

No. There is currently no recommended booster dose of MenB vaccine for any group.

Should persons with continued high risk of meningococcal disease receive additional doses of meningococcal vaccine beyond the 3- or 5-year booster?

Yes, people should receive additional booster doses (every 5 years) if they continue to be at highest risk for meningococcal infection.

HUMAN PAPILLOMAVIRUS

Did you know that:

- Infection with human papillomavirus (HPV) is universal among humans (both females and males).
- The vast majority of US teenagers are not aware that a single sexual contact with an infected partner with or without a visible lesion can spread HPV.
- Every 20 minutes in the United States a person acquires an infection with HPV.
- In the USA, among girls 14 to 19 years old, HPV incidence dropped by nearly two-thirds from 11.5% to 4.3% since the introduction of HPV vaccines in 2006. For women 20 to 24 the rate was down slightly more than one-third from 18.5% to 12.1%.

In the United States, HPV will infect 80% of sexually active males and females in their lifetime. According to the CDC, there are approximately 14 million new genital HPV infections in the United States each year, half of which occur in people ages 15 to 24 years. For most people, HPV clears spontaneously, but for those who do not clear the virus, infection can lead to significant cancers and other diseases in men and women. There is no way to predict who in the population will clear the virus, although, the oncogenic types are more likely to persist and lead to the development of malignancy than the benign types.

Human papillomavirus (HPV) causes a range of disease manifestations including: cutaneous non-genital warts of the skin (e.g., common skin warts, plantar warts, flat warts, filiform warts), mucous membranes (e.g., anogenital, oral, nasal, and conjunctival areas), and the respiratory tract (e.g., respiratory papillomatosis).

It also is associated with cervical, anogenital, and oropharyngeal dysplasias (precancers) and cancers. There are over 100 different serotypes of HPV that have been identified. These serotypes are subdivided into high-risk, oncogenic, serotypes and low-risk, non-oncogenic serotypes. The most common high-risk serotypes include types 16, 18, 31, 33, 35, 39, 45, 51, 52, 56, 58, 59, 68, 69, 73, 82, which account for 98% of all cervical cancers. Serotypes 16 and 18 account for 70% of all cervical cancers and the vast majority of other anogenital cancers. The most common low-risk serotypes include types 6, 11, 40, 42, 43, 44, 54, with serotypes 6 and 11 accounting for 90% of all external anogenital warts.

Transmission

Transmission takes place person to person by close contact. Nongenital warts are acquired through contact with HPV and minor trauma to the skin. Anogenital HPV infection is the most common sexually transmitted infection in the United States. Most infections are subclinical and resolve spontaneously within 2 years. Persistent infection with high-risk types of HPV is associated with development of cervical, vulvar, vaginal, penile, anal, and oropharyngeal cancers. In the case of respiratory papillomatosis, infection is transmitted to an infant through the birth canal during delivery by aspiration of infectious secretions. The finding of genital warts or laryngeal lesions in young children should raise the suspicion of child abuse.

Incubation period

Incubation period is unknown but is estimated to range from 3 months to 10 years.

Prevention

Condoms, both male and female provide some protection but as the male condom only covers the shaft of the penis, there is still the potential for contact and spread from the anogenital area. Female condoms that cover much of the anogenital area and the entire vagina should provide more protection; however, the usage of female condoms is not widespread or even advertised significantly.

The best protection is provided by HPV vaccines.

Postexposure

a. HPV vaccine—there are three vaccines currently licensed in United States:

i. HPV4 (contains serotypes 6/11/16/18)—licensed for use in *both* girls and boys 9 through 26 years of age for the prevention of cervical intraepithelial neoplasia (CINs), vulvar intraepithelial neoplasia (VIN), vaginal intraepithelial neoplasia (VAIN), cervical, vulvar, vaginal cancers, anal intraepithelial neoplasia (AIN), anal cancers, and genital warts. It is given as a 3-dose intramuscular series at 0, 1 to 2, and 6 months.

ii. HPV2 (contains serotypes 16/18)—licensed for use in girls 10 through 25 years of age for the prevention of CIN1, 2, 3; cervical AIS; and cervical cancer. It is given as a 3-dose intramuscular series at 0, 1, and 6 months.

iii. HPV9 (contains the 4 serotypes in HPV4 6/11/16/18 plus 5 additional serotypes 31, 33, 45, 52, 58). It is licensed for use in *both* females and males ages 9–25, and is replacing HPV-4. It is given as a 3 dose intramuscular series at 0, 1–2, and 6 months or 2 dose intramuscular series at 0 and 6 months for adolescents 11 to 14 years of age. Effectiveness is expected to be over 90% worldwide.

    iv. HPV vaccine is still recommended to be given even after onset of sexual activity and if HPV positive since very unlikely to be infected with more than one serotype.

    v. These vaccines are *not* therapeutic vaccines and are not useful in treating any specific HPV-related conditions.

Preexposure

  a. HPV vaccines—the best time to administer is prior to the onset of sexual activity. It is not prudent to give the vaccine based on perceived risk, since it is not possible to predict onset of sexual activity in any patient. In multiple studies in New Zealand, Australia, and the United States, there was no increased sexual activity related to immunizing adolescents with HPV vaccine.

    i. HPV4 (contains serotypes 6/11/16/18)—licensed for use in *both* girls and boys 9 through 26 years of age for the prevention of cervical CINs, vulvar intraepithelial neoplasia (VIN), vaginal intraepithelial neoplasia (VAIN), anal cancers, and genital warts. It is given as a 3-dose intramuscular series at 0, 1 to 2, and 6 months.

    ii. HPV2 (contains serotypes 16/18)—licensed for use in girls 10 through 25 years of age for the prevention of CIN 1, 2, 3; cervical AIS; and cervical cancer. It is given as a 3-dose intramuscular series at 0, 1, and 6 months.

    iii. HPV9 (contains the 4 serotypes in HPV4 6/11/16/18 plus 5 additional serotypes 31, 33, 45, 52, 58). Licensed for use in both females and males ages 9–25, and is replacing HPV-4. It is given as a 3-dose intramuscular series at 0, 1–2, and 6 months or 0 and 6 months for the 2 dose series in adolescents 11 to 14 years of age.

    iv. Vaccines are *not* to be used as therapeutic vaccines.

Immunogenicity

a. All HPV vaccines are 98% to 100% effective for the prevention of cervical precancers due to vaccine serotypes.
b. HPV4 and HPV9 are 98% to 100% effective for the prevention of VIN and VAIN.
c. HPV4 and HPV9 are 90% effective for the prevention of genital warts and anal cancers.

Vaccination rates in females and males 13 to 17 years of age in the United States remain around 39.7% and 21.6% respectively for receiving all 3 doses. Young patients are strongly encouraged to be vaccinated and parents should be strongly encouraged to have their children vaccinated. The emphasis must be "this is a cancer vaccine," not a "sexual activity" vaccine. The recommendation of the health-care provider is the most important factor in a patient or parent's acceptance of the vaccination.

Duration of immunity

Duration is at least 12 years.

Contraindications and precautions to HPV vaccine

Contraindications
1. Severe allergic reaction (e.g., anaphylaxis) after a previous dose or to a vaccine component
2. HPV4 and HPV9—severe allergic reaction (e.g., anaphylaxis) to yeast
3. HPV2—severe allergic reaction (e.g., anaphylaxis) to latex

Precautions
1. Moderate or severe acute illness with or without fever
2. Pregnancy

Frequently asked questions

If a person was vaccinated at age 11 years and completed the 3-dose series, and is now aged 20 years and sexually active, should she receive a booster dose of vaccine?
NO. Long-term studies have shown no loss of efficacy at least 13 years after the first series of vaccinations.

Should individuals who have completed a 3-dose series of HPV2 or HPV4 receive a booster dose or be revaccinated with a 3-dose series of HPV9?
At this time, there are no recommendations for a booster dose of vaccine or revaccination with HPV9. There are data that indicate revaccination with HPV9 after a series of HPV4 is safe. Clinicians should decide if the benefit of immunity against 5 additional oncogenic strains of HPV is justified for their patients.

If a patient received 1 or 2 doses and has not completed the 3-dose series, should the series be restarted?
NO. Even if a long period of time has passed since the last vaccine dose, the series should not be restarted but should be resumed where it was left off and can be completed at any time. However, if multiple doses are needed, the timing between doses cannot be shortened.

Should HPV9 be used in males ages 16 to 26 years, given that current FDA licensure is for males 9 to 15 years of age?
Although HPV9 vaccine was initially licensed for use in males aged 9 to 15 years, the CDC ACIP and the AAP recommend that this vaccine be used in males through age 21 years routinely and in high-risk males age 21 to 26 years old. To arrive at this off-label male recommendation, the CDC ACIP reviewed data that was not yet available during

the FDA licensure process. This has now been submitted for FDA review.

Will giving HPV vaccination encourage sexual activity in my teenage child?
No. Multiple studies have shown no difference in the initiation of sexual activity in adolescents who have or not received the HPV vaccine. These studies used STD incidence, use of contraception, pregnancy and abortion rates in determining the lack of differences in the 2 groups.

If a woman becomes pregnant and has received only 1 or 2 doses of HPV vaccine can she complete the series during the pregnancy?
No. Even though HPV vaccine poses no risk to the fetus, the doses should be delayed until after the pregnancy. She may receive the vaccine even if she is breast feeding.

Is HPV vaccine effective for patients over the age of 26 years?
HPV vaccine has been tested in patients up to age 45 years, and although there is an immune response, it is less robust than what occurs in younger patients. Patients could receive the vaccine off label, however, insurance would probably not pay for the vaccine.

If a patient has received 1 or 2 doses of HPV2 or HPV4 vaccine, can the patient complete the series with HPV9?
Yes. Any available HPV vaccine may be used to continue to complete the series for females. HPV4 or HPV9 can be used to continue or complete the series for males. However, receiving fewer than 3 doses of HPV4 or HPV9 may provide less

protection against genital warts caused by HPV types 6 and 11 than the usual 3-dose series. There are no data on the efficacy of the 5 additional HPV types included in HPV9 if the person receives fewer than 3 doses.

Can the HPV vaccine damage a woman's ovaries?

No. The CDC and FDA have found no evidence that HPV vaccine is associated with premature ovarian failure. There has also been no evidence of amenorrhea or irregular menses in women who have received the vaccine.

Why is HPV vaccine recommended if Pap tests can detect cervical cancer?

Pap tests are effective screening tests and can detect precancerous changes before progression to cancer. But the vaccine actually prevents cancer in the first place, and Pap tests are not perfect (overall 50% sensitivity), and not all women get tested as often as recommended.

Should women still have Pap tests done after receiving HPV vaccine?

Yes. Although the HPV9 vaccine protects against over 90% of the cancer producing HPV viruses, many women have received either the HPV2 or HPV4 vaccines which protect against approximately 70% of oncogenic virus types. Pap screening recommendations may well change as a higher percentage of women are vaccinated.

Do women and men whose sexual orientation is same sex need HPV vaccine?

Yes. HPV vaccine is recommended for females and males regardless of their sexual orientation.

Is there an accelerated vaccination schedule to complete the HPV vaccine series?

No. There is no accelerated schedule for completing the HPV vaccine series. The recommended schedule of 0, 1–2, and 6 months or 0 and 6 months (adolescents 11 to 14 years of age) should be followed.

If HPV vaccine is inadvertently given subcutaneously instead of intramuscularly, does the dose need to be repeated?

Yes. No data exist on the efficacy or safety of HPV vaccine given by the subcutaneous route, therefore, the CDC and the manufacturers recommend that a dose of HPV vaccine given by any route other than intramuscular should be repeated. There is no minimum interval between the invalid subcutaneous dose and the repeat dose.

HAEMOPHILUS INFLUENZAE TYPE B (HIB) DISEASE

Did you know that:

- Before the availability of Hib conjugate vaccine, each year in the United States about 20,000 children under 5 years of age got Hib disease, and 3% to 6% died from their disease.
- The bacteria was first isolated by Pfeiffer from the sputum of patients in 1892 during an outbreak of influenza, and it was proposed that there was a causal association between the bacteria and the clinical syndrome of influenza.

Haemophilus influenzae type b (Hib) is a pleomorphic gram-negative coccobacillus. It may cause a variety of different infections including pneumonia, bacteremia, meningitis, epiglottis, septic arthritis, osteomyelitis, cellulitis, otitis media, purulent pericarditis, endocarditis, endophthalmitis, peritonitis and gangrene. Before the introduction of effective Hib conjugate vaccines (before 1990), Hib was the most common cause of bacterial meningitis in children in the United States. There were 20,000 cases a year of invasive disease with the peak age of infections occurring in infants between 6 and 18 months of age. Non-type b encapsulated strains cause disease similar to type b infections. Nontypeable strains commonly cause infections of the respiratory tract (e.g., otitis media, sinusitis, pneumonia, and conjunctivitis). Less commonly, these strains may be the cause of bacteremia, meningitis, chorioamnionitis, and neonatal sepsis.

Unimmunized children ≤4 years of age are at increased risk of invasive Hib disease. Other risk factors that predispose to invasive disease in all ages include: sickle cell disease, asplenia, human immunodeficiency virus (HIV) infection, certain immunodeficiency syndromes and malignant neoplasms. Historically, invasive Hib disease was more common in boys; black, Alaskan Native, Apache, and Navajo children; daycare attendees; children living in crowded conditions; and children who were not breastfed. Since the introduction of Hib conjugate vaccines in the United States, the incidence of invasive Hib disease has decreased by 99%. Currently, invasive disease occurs primarily in underimmunized children and among infants too young to have completed the primary immunization series. Hib remains a major pathogen in many resource-limited countries where Hib vaccine is not routinely available. In the United States, non-typeable *H. influenzae* now causes the majority of invasive disease in all age groups.

Transmission

The major reservoir of Hib is young infants and toddlers who carry the organism in the upper respiratory tract, which is the nature habitat of *H. influenzae* in humans. Transmission is person-to-person by inhalation of respiratory tract droplets or by direct contact with infected respiratory tract secretions. In neonates, infection is acquired intrapartum by aspiration of amniotic fluid or by contact with genital tract secretions containing the organism. Pharyngeal colonization by *H. influenzae* is common, especially with nontypeable and non-type b capsular types.

Incubation period

Unknown

Prevention is available only for Hib

Post-exposure
Careful observation of exposed, unimmunized, or incompletely immunized children who are household, childcare, or nursery school contacts of patients with invasive Hib disease is essential.

   a. Chemoprophylaxis—the risk of invasive Hib disease is increased among unimmunized, or incompletely immunized household contacts younger than 4 years of age. Rifampin (20 mg/kg, max dose 600 mg—given once a day for 4 days) eradicates Hib from the pharynx in about 95% of carriers and decreases the risk of secondary invasive infection in exposed household contacts. Nursery and childcare center contacts under 4 years of age may also be at increased risk of secondary disease. The following are indications for rifampin chemoprophylaxis for contacts of index cases of invasive Hib disease.
   • For all household contacts (defined as people living with the index patient or nonresidents who spend 4 or more

hours with the index patient for at least 5 of the 7 days preceding the day of hospital admission) in the following circumstances:

- household with at least 1 contact younger that 4 years of age who is unimmunized or incompletely immunized
- household with a child younger than 12 months of age who has not completed the primary Hib series
- household with a contact who is an immunocompromised child, regardless of that child's Hib immunization status
- for preschool and childcare contacts when 2 or more cases of Hib invasive disease have occurred within 60 days
- for index patient, if younger than 2 years of age or member of household with a susceptible contact and **treated with a regimen other than ceftriaxone or cefotaxime**, chemoprophylaxis is provided just before hospital discharge

b. Hib vaccine—in addition to chemoprophylaxis, unimmunized or incompletely immunized children should receive a dose of Hib vaccine and should be scheduled for completion of the recommended age-specific immunization schedule.

Preexposure

a. Hib vaccine—vaccine is given intramuscularly

   i. Primary series—depending on the vaccine used, the recommended primary series consists of 3 doses given at 2, 4, and 6 months of age (DTaP-IPV/PRP-T), or 2 doses given at 2 and 4 months of age (PRP-OMP, PRP-OMP-HepB). If PRP-OMP vaccine is **not administered** as both doses in the primary series, a **third dose of Hib conjugate vaccine** is **needed** to complete the primary series.

   ii. Booster dose—recommended to be given at 12 through 15 months of age.

Contraindications and Precautions for Hib vaccine

Contraindications
1. Severe allergic reaction (e.g., anaphylaxis) after a previous dose or to a vaccine component.
2. Age younger than 6 weeks.

Precautions
Moderate or severe acute illness with or without fever

Efficacy

Efficacy is 98% to 100% against Hib.

Frequently asked questions

Can all the licensed Hib-containing vaccines be used interchangeably?
Yes, but there is one exception. The GSK monovalent product (Hiberix) is only licensed for the booster dose of vaccine.

If Hiberix is inadvertently given as some or all of the doses of the primary Hib vaccine series, do the doses need to be repeated?
No, the administered doses count and *do not* need to be re-administered with another Hib vaccine.

If an infant received one dose of Hib at 4 months of age, and another at 16 months of age, do they need any additional doses of Hib vaccine?
No, if an infant receives a dose of Hib vaccine at 15 months of age or older, they do not need any further Hib vaccine doses regardless of the number of doses received before 15 months of age.

If a 4-year-old patient received dose #3 of Hib vaccine at 6 months of age, does the child need a fourth dose of Hib?

Yes, all children less than 5 years of age need at least one dose of Hib vaccine on or after the first birthday. The last dose should be separated from the previous dose by at least 2 months.

The booster dose of Hib vaccine is recommended to be given at 12 to 15 months of age. If a patient received their first dose of Hib vaccine at 12 months of age, is it necessary to administer the booster dose 2 months later?

If the child received a primary series (2 or 3 doses) of Hib vaccine in the first year of life, then the final (booster) dose of the series may be given as early as 12 months, provided at least 2 months have passed since the last dose. An unvaccinated 12- to 14-month-old child should receive one dose of Hib vaccine as the primary series, and a booster dose 2 months later. Unvaccinated children 15 to 59 months of age need only a single dose of any licensed conjugate Hib vaccine.

Does an 8-year old who does not have a record of ever receiving Hib vaccine need a dose?

The CDC does not recommend routine Hib vaccination of healthy children 59 months or older, even if they have no prior history of receiving Hib vaccination.

Which adults should receive a dose of Hib vaccine?

Hib vaccine is recommended for adults with sickle cell disease, leukemia, HIV infection, and persons with functional or anatomic asplenia if they have not previously received Hib vaccine. A standard pediatric dose of any Hib vaccine may be used. Hib vaccine is not routinely recommended for healthy adults 19 years of age and older.

When should Hib vaccine be administered to a person having a splenectomy?
When elective splenectomy is planned, vaccination with pneumococcal, meningococcal, and Hib vaccines should be administered at least 2 weeks prior to the surgery, if possible. If the vaccines are not administered before surgery, they should be administered as soon as the person's condition stabilizes post-operatively.

POLIOVIRUS INFECTIONS

Did you know that:

- None of the 3 strains of wild poliovirus can survive outside the human body for very long and will die out if the virus can't find an unvaccinated person to infect.
- Franklin D. Roosevelt, the thirty-second president of the United States, contracted paralytic polio at the age of 39, resulting in partial paralysis of his legs and the inability to walk without the aid of crutches, leg braces, or a wheelchair.
- In addition to Franklin Delano Roosevelt, a well-known polio survivor; others include science fiction writer Arthur C. Clarke, artist Frida Kahlo, golfer Jack Nicklaus, swimmer (and actor) Johnny Weissmuller, actors Mia Farrow and Alan Alda, and singer/songwriters Neil Young and Joni Mitchell.
- Poliomyelitis has affected humankind since ancient times. An Egyptian stele from the 18th dynasty (1403 to 1365 BC) depicts a crippled young man with a withered and

shortened right leg, with his foot held in a typical equinus position characteristic of flaccid paralysis.

- In the prevaccine era, poliomyelitis was the leading cause of permanent disability. It was a feared disease because it could strike anyone, and no means existed to protect oneself or one's children.
- Epidemic poliomyelitis in the early 20th century was associated with a case fatality rate of 27.1%.
- The first iron lung was constructed in 1928 and its widespread use in the 1930s and 1940s rapidly decreased the case fatality rate of bulbar forms of poliomyelitis.
- The game Candy Land was invented in 1948 by a patient trying to cheer up kids in a polio ward.
- Polio can be completely eradicated.

Polioviruses are group C enteroviruses that consist of serotypes 1, 2, and 3. Poliovirus infections occur only in humans. About 72% of poliovirus infections in susceptible children are asymptomatic. A non-specific febrile illness with low-grade fever and sore throat occurs in 24% of people who become infected. Aseptic meningitis (pleocytosis with a lymphocytic predominance), sometimes with paresthesias occurs in 1% to 5% of patients a few days after the minor illness has resolved. Paralytic polio occurs in less than 1% of infected persons. There is the rapid onset of asymmetric acute flaccid paralysis with areflexia of the involved limb and residual paralytic disease involving the motor neurons that occurs in approximately two-thirds of people with acute motor neuron disease. Cranial nerve involvement and paralysis of respiratory tract muscles can occur.

Adults who contracted paralytic poliomyelitis during childhood may develop the non-infectious post-polio syndrome 15 to 40 years later. Post-polio syndrome is characterized by slow and irreversible exacerbation of weakness most likely occurring in those muscle groups involved during the original infection. Muscle and joint pain are common. Studies estimate the risk of post-polio syndrome in poliomyelitis survivors to be 25% to 40%.

No cases of polio have originated in the United States since 1979; the last case of wild-type polio in a US resident traveling abroad occurred in 1986, and the last imported case of polio in the United States occurred in 1993. Globally, polio cases have decreased by over 99% since 1988 due to a concerted global effort to eradicate the disease. In 1994 the World Health Organization (WHO) Region of the Americas was certified polio-free, followed by the WHO Western Pacific Region in 2000, the WHO European Region in June 2002, and the WHO South East Asian Region in 2014. Of the three types of wild poliovirus, type 2 wild poliovirus transmission has been successfully eradicated since 1999. In 2016 only 2 countries in the world continue to have endemic circulating wildtype poliovirus—Afghanistan, and Pakistan, down from 125 in 1988. However, as long as wildtype poliovirus continues to circulate, children in all countries are at risk of contracting polio.

Transmission

Spread is by the fecal, oral, and respiratory routes. Infection is more common in infants and young children and occurs at an earlier age among children living in poor hygienic conditions. Communicability of poliovirus is greatest shortly before and after the onset of clinical disease, when the virus is present in the throat and is excreted in high concentration in the feces. Virus persists in the throat for approximately 2 weeks after onset of illness and is excreted in the feces for 3 to 6 weeks. Patients are potentially contagious as long as fecal excretion persists.

Incubation period

For nonparalytic polio, the incubation period is 3 to 6 days. For the onset of paralysis in paralytic poliomyelitis, the incubation period is usually 7 to 21 days.

Prevention

Preexposure prophylaxis

a. Inactivated polio vaccine (IPV)—four doses of IPV vaccine are recommended for routine immunization of all infants and children.

   i. The first 2 doses of the 4-dose vaccine series should be given at 2-month intervals beginning at 2 months of age (2 mo, 4 mo). The third dose is recommended to be given at 6 through 18 months of age. A fourth and final dose in the series should be administered at 4 years of age or older regardless of the number of previous doses and at a minimum interval of 6 months from the third dose. If a child misses an IPV dose at 4 through 6 years of age, the child should receive a booster dose as soon as feasible.

   ii. Most adults living in the United States are presumed to be immune as a result of previous immunization. However, immunization is recommended for certain adults who are a greater risk of exposure to wild-type polioviruses than the general population, including the following:
      • travelers to areas or countries where poliomyelitis is or may be epidemic or endemic
      • laboratory workers handling specimens that may contain wild-type polioviruses

- health-care personnel in close contact with patients who may be excreting wild-type polioviruses

For unimmunized or incompletely immunized adults, primary immunization with IPV vaccine is recommended as a series of 3 doses. Two doses of IPV vaccine should be given at intervals of 1 to 2 months (4 to 8 weeks); a third dose is given 6 to 12 months after the second dose. If 3 doses of IPV cannot be administered within the recommended intervals before protection is needed, the following alternatives are recommended:

- If >8 weeks are available before protection is needed, 3 doses of IPV should be administered ≥4 weeks apart.
- If <8 weeks but >4 weeks are available before protection is needed, 2 doses of IPV should be administered ≥4 weeks apart.
- If <4 weeks are available before protection is needed, a single dose of IPV is recommended.

Vaccine efficacy

Both inactivated polio vaccine (IPV) and oral live, attenuated polio vaccine (OPV) are highly immunogenic and effective in preventing poliomyelitis. IPV is the only polio vaccine available in the United States. After 2 doses of IPV, greater than 95% of recipients seroconvert to the 3 polio serotypes contained in the vaccine. After 3 doses, seroconversion is seen in 99% to 100% of vaccine recipients.

Duration of immunity

At least 18 years after a 3-dose series of vaccine.

Contraindications and precautions for polio vaccine

Contraindications

Vaccine is contraindicated for people who have experienced an anaphylactic reaction after a previous dose of IPV vaccine or to streptomycin, neomycin, or polymyxin B.

Precautions

1. Moderate or severe acute illness with or without fever
2. Pregnancy

Frequently asked questions

If there is no longer any polio in the Western Hemisphere, why do we still recommend universal polio vaccination?
If polio vaccination were discontinued in the United States, there would be millions of susceptible children within a year. Since wild polio infection still occurs in the world, the virus could be imported and an epidemic could result.

After what age is routine polio vaccine no longer recommended?
Routine polio vaccination is not recommended for persons 18 years of age and older who reside in the United States.

Exceptions would include adults at risk for coming into contact with polio virus: traveling in polio-endemic areas of the world (currently Afghanistan or Pakistan), working in a laboratory and handling specimens that might contain polio-viruses, and those who may have close contact with someone who could be infected with poliovirus.

Is vaccine-derived poliovirus a risk in the United States?

Vaccine-derived poliovirus (VDPV) is a strain of poliovirus that was initially contained in OPV and that has mutated over time and behaves more like the wild-type virus. These strains may be transmitted to unvaccinated persons and cause illness, including paralytic poliomyelitis—indistinguishable from the illness caused by wild-type poliovirus. VDPV can cause outbreaks in countries where vaccine coverage with OPV is low. Because OPV has not been used in the United States since 2000 and vaccine coverage with IPV is high, the risk of VDPV in the United States is very low. It would be possible for an unvaccinated person to acquire VDPV from some who recently received live oral vaccine in another country.

How long is oral polio vaccine virus shed in the stool after the dose?

OPV may be shed in the stool for up to 6 weeks, but can be longer in immunosuppressed individuals. Viral shedding in the stool is generally longest following the first dose and is generally shorter with each subsequent dose.

A 4-year-old who is entering pre-K has a vaccination record that shows that they received 4 doses of IPV given at 2 months, 4 months, 6 months, and 2 years of age. Does this child need a booster dose of vaccine?

Yes. The current recommendations are that a child receive 4 doses of IPV vaccine with the last dose being given on or after the fourth birthday.

If a 10-year-old child adopted from another country received three doses of oral polio vaccine (OPV) before their first birthday, should they receive an additional dose of inactivated poliovirus vaccine (IPV)?

Yes. The patient should receive a dose of IPV now. The final dose of the polio vaccine series should be received on or after the fourth birthday, regardless of the number of doses received prior to the fourth birthday.

What polio vaccination schedule should be used for older children who have not completed their IPV series?

The schedule for polio vaccination for unvaccinated or under-vaccinated older children through age 17 years is a total of 3 doses of IPV: 2 doses of IPV separated by 4 to 8 weeks, and a third dose 6 to 12 months after the second dose. Polio vaccine is not routinely administered to persons 18 years of age and older.

Should adults get vaccinated against polio if they are traveling to a high-risk area where polio still occurs?

If an adult at increased risk previously received only one or two doses or polio vaccine (either OPV or IPV), they should receive the remaining dose(s) of IPV regardless of the interval since the last polio vaccine dose. If the at risk adult previously completed a primary course of polio vaccine (three of more doses of OPV or IPV), they may be given another dose of IPV to ensure protection. Only "one" booster dose of polio vaccine in a person's lifetime is recommended. It is not necessary to administer a booster dose each time a person travels to an area where polio may be occurring.

Should an adult, who was diagnosed with polio as a child with some residual effects that now will be traveling to a

high-risk area where polio still occurs, be vaccinated with polio vaccine even though they had polio in the past?
Immunity to one of the serotypes of polio does not produce significant immunity to the other serotypes. A history of having recovered from polio disease should not be considered evidence of immunity to polio. In this situation it is appropriate to vaccinate this person with a dose of IPV if they are traveling to a high-risk area.

A 22-year-old patient has been accepted to a medical school that requires polio vaccine for all the students. The patient has 2 documented doses of OPV vaccine as a child, then received a dose of IPV upon college entry at age 18 years. How many additional doses of IPV should this patient receive to complete the series and on what schedule?
Persons who receive a mixed series of OPV and IPV should receive a total of 4 doses of vaccine. The dose of IPV can be counted as the third dose in the primary series. The minimum interval between the third and last doses in the polio vaccination series is 6 months; therefore, the final dose in the series should be administered 6 months or greater after the last IPV dose.

ROTAVIRUS INFECTIONS

Did you know that:

- Worldwide, rotavirus is estimated to cause 450,000 to 600,000 deaths in children each year, which is approximately 20 to 25% of the estimated 1.9 million annual deaths from diarrhea.

- Rotavirus diarrheal illness causes 1,200 to 1,600 deaths per day in developing countries.
- Fluid loss from severe rotavirus diarrhea in an infant can be as much as 20 ml/Kg per hour.

Rotaviruses are segmented, double-stranded RNA viruses with at least 7 distinct antigenic groups (A through G). Group A viruses are the major causes of rotavirus diarrhea worldwide. Serotyping is based on the 2 surface proteins, VP7 glycoprotein (G) and VP4 protease-cleaved hemagglutinin (P). Prior to introduction of the rotavirus vaccine, G types 1 through 4 and 9 and P types 1A and 1B were the most common in the United States. Rotavirus infection is the leading cause of severe acute diarrhea among young children worldwide. In the United States, prior to the introduction of rotavirus vaccine in 2006, rotavirus caused an estimated 20 to 60 deaths, 55,000 to 70,000 hospitalizations, 205,000 to 272,000 emergency department visits, and 410,000 outpatient visits annually. Nearly every child in the United States was infected with rotavirus by 5 years of age and most developed gastroenteritis. Rotavirus was responsible for 5%–10% of all gastroenteritis episodes among children less than 5 years of age in the United States.

Infection begins with the acute onset of fever and vomiting followed 24 to 48 hours later by watery diarrhea. Symptoms generally persists for 3 to 8 days. In moderate to severe cases, dehydration, electrolyte abnormalities, and acidosis may occur. The epidemiology of rotavirus disease in the United States has changed dramatically since rotavirus vaccines became available in 2006. The overall burden of rotavirus disease has significantly declined. In the first 2 years after the RV5 vaccine became available, ER visits and hospitalizations for rotavirus decreased by 85% (estimated 40,000 to 60,000 fewer gastroenteritis hospitalizations among children younger than 5 years of age.) There were also substantial reductions in office visits for gastroenteritis during this time period.

Transmission

Believed to be by the fecal-oral route. Rotavirus can be found on toys and hard surfaces in child-care centers, indicating that fomites may also serve as a mechanism of transmission. Respiratory transmission may play a minor role in disease transmission.

Incubation period

1 to 3 days

Prevention

Preexposure

a. Rotavirus vaccine—there are 2 rotavirus vaccines licensed for use among infants in the United States (Table 16). In February 2006, a live, oral human-bovine reassortant pentavalent rotavirus vaccine (RV5) was licensed as a 3-dose series for use among infants in the United States. In April 2008, a live, oral human attenuated monovalent rotavirus vaccine (RV1) was licensed as a 2-dose series for infants in the United States. Vaccine is administered orally.

   i. Rotavirus vaccine can be administered concurrently with other childhood vaccines.

   ii. Preterm infants may be immunized if at least 6 weeks of postnatal age and are clinically stable. They should be immunized on the same schedule and with the same precautions recommended for full-term infants. The

Table 16 ORAL ROTAVIRUS VACCINES

Recommendation for Use	RV5 (RotaTeq—Merck)	RV1 (Rotarix—GSK)
Number of doses in the series	3	2
Recommended ages for doses	2, 4, and 6 months of age	2 and 4 months of age
Minimum age for first dose	6 weeks of age	6 weeks of age
Maximum age for first dose	14 weeks, 6 days of age	14 weeks, 6 days of age
Minimum interval between doses	4 weeks	4 weeks
Maximum age for last dose	8 months, 0 days of age	8 months, 0 days of age

first dose of the vaccine should be given at the time of discharge or after the infant has been discharged from the nursery.

iii. Breastfeeding infants should be immunized according to the same schedule as non-breastfed infants.

iv. Infants who have had rotavirus gastroenteritis before receiving the full series of rotavirus immunization should begin or complete the schedule following the standard age and interval recommendations.

Vaccine contraindications

1. Rotavirus vaccine should *not* be given to infants who have a history of a severe allergic reaction (e.g., anaphylaxis) after a previous dose of rotavirus vaccine or to a vaccine component. Latex rubber is contained in the RV1 vaccine oral applicator, so infants with a severe allergy to latex (e.g., anaphylaxis) should not receive RV1.

2. Severe combined immunodeficiency (SCID) and a history of intussusception are contraindications for use of both RV1 and RV5 rotavirus vaccines.

Vaccine efficacy

a. RV5—effectiveness after 3-dose series ranges from 96% to 100% against severe rotavirus disease, 78% to 100% against disease requiring hospitalization and 96% in preventing disease requiring an outpatient visit

b. RV1—effectiveness after 2-dose series ranges from 76% to 89% against rotavirus disease requiring hospitalization and 50% in preventing disease requiring an outpatient visit

Frequently asked questions

How long is a person with rotavirus diarrhea contagious?
Infected persons shed large quantities of virus in their stool beginning 2 days before the onset of diarrhea and for up to 10 days after onset of symptoms. Rotavirus may be detected in the stool of persons with immune deficiency for more than 30 days after infection.

Can a person get rotavirus disease more than once?
Yes. A person may develop rotavirus disease more than once because there are many different rotavirus types, but second infections tend to be less severe than the first infections. After a single natural infection, 40% of children are protected against a subsequent rotavirus illness. Persons of all ages can get repeated rotavirus infections, but symptoms may be mild or not occur at all in repeat infections.

Can adults be infected with rotavirus?

Yes. Rotavirus infection of adults is usually asymptomatic but may cause diarrheal illness. Outbreaks of diarrheal illness caused by rotavirus have been reported, especially among elderly persons living in retirement communities and nursing homes.

Should an infant who has already been infected with rotavirus still be vaccinated?

Yes. Infants who have recovered from a rotavirus infection may not be immune to all of the virus types present in the vaccine. So infants who have previously had rotavirus disease should still complete the vaccine series if they can do so by age 8 months.

If it is unknown which rotavirus vaccine an infant previously received, how should the vaccine schedule be completed?

If the product used for a previous dose is unknown, and the infant is at an age when the vaccine can still be administered, a total of 3 doses of rotavirus vaccine should be given. All doses of vaccine should be administered by age 8 months and 0 days.

If the first dose of rotavirus vaccine is inadvertently given to an infant age 15 weeks and older, should the vaccine series be continued?

Infants for whom the first dose of rotavirus vaccine was inadvertently administered at age 15 weeks or older should receive the remaining doses of the series at the routinely recommended intervals. The timing of the first dose should not affect the safety and efficacy of the remaining doses. Rotavirus vaccine should not be given after 8 months 0 days even if the series is incomplete.

In the situation where an infant received the first dose of rotavirus vaccine but got laboratory confirmed rotavirus disease prior to the second vaccine dose, should the infant complete the vaccine series?

CDC recommends that infants who have had rotavirus gastroenteritis before receiving the full series of rotavirus vaccination should still start or complete the schedule according to the age and interval recommendations since the initial rotavirus infection might provide only partial protection against subsequent rotavirus disease.

If an infant regurgitates or vomits during or after rotavirus vaccine administration, should the dose be repeated?

No—if an infant spits, regurgitates, or vomits during or after rotavirus vaccine has been administered, the dose should not be repeated. The next dose of vaccine should be administered at the appropriate interval.

Can an infant receive rotavirus vaccine if there are pregnant or immunocompromised individuals that live in the same household?

Infants living in households with pregnant women or immunocompromised people *can* be immunized with rotavirus vaccine. Transmission of vaccine virus strains from vaccines to unimmunized contacts is uncommon.

Table 17 CONTRADICTIONS AND PRECAUTIONS FOR COMMONLY USED VACCINES

Vaccine	Contraindications	Precautions
For **all** vaccines	Severe allergic reaction (e.g., anaphylaxis) after a previous dose or to a vaccine component	Moderate or severe acute illness with or without fever

In addition to the above, addition contraindications and precautions for specific vaccines

Vaccine	Contraindications	Precautions
Diphtheria, tetanus, pertussis (DTaP, DTP) Tetanus, diphtheria, pertussis (Tdap) Tetanus, diphtheria (DT, Td)	For pertussis containing vaccines: encephalopathy (e.g., coma, decreased level of consciousness, prolonged seizures) not attributable to another identifiable cause within 7 days of administration of a previous dose of DTP, DTaP, or Tdap	• Guillain-Barré Syndrome (GBS) within 6 weeks after a previous dose of tetanus toxoid-containing vaccine • History of Arthus-type hypersensitivity reactions after a previous dose of tetanus or diphtheria toxoid-containing vaccine; defer vaccination until at least 10 years have elapsed since the last tetanus-toxoid-containing vaccine • For pertussis-containing vaccines: progressive or unstable neurologic disorder (including infantile spasms for DTaP), uncontrolled seizures, or

Table 17 CONTINUED

Vaccine	Contraindications	Precautions
		progressive encephalopathy until a treatment regimen has been established and the condition has stabilized
		For DTaP/DTP only:
		• Temperature of 105°F or higher (40.5°C or higher) within 48 hours after vaccination with a previous dose of DTP/DTaP
		• Collapse or shocklike state (i.e., hypotonic hyporesponsive episode) within 48 hours after receiving a previous dose of DTP/DTaP
		• Seizure within 3 days after receiving a previous dose of DTP/DTaP
		• Persistent, inconsolable crying lasting 3 or more hours within 48 hours after receiving a previous dose of DTP/DTaP
Haemophilus influenzae Type b (Hib)	Age younger than 6 weeks	—
Hepatitis B	—	Infants weighing less than 2000 grams (4 lbs, 6.4 oz)

(*continued*)

Table 17 CONTINUED

Vaccine	Contraindications	Precautions
Human papillomavirus (HPV)	• Severe allergic reaction (e.g. anaphylaxis) to yeast—HPV4, HPV9 • Severe allergic reaction (e.g. anaphylaxis) to latex—HPV2	Pregnancy
Inactivated poliovirus vaccine (IPV)	—	Pregnancy
Influenza, inactivated injectable (IIV)	Severe allergic reaction (e.g., anaphylaxis) to prior dose of vaccine or to vaccine component	• History of Guillain-Barré syndrome (GBS) within 6 weeks of previous influenza vaccination • Persons who experience only hives with exposure to eggs may receive recombinant influenza vaccine (RIV) or, with additional safety precautions, IIV.
Influenza, recombinant (RIV)—Flublok	Severe allergic reaction (e.g., anaphylaxis) after a previous dose or to a vaccine component, RIV does not contain any egg protein, thimerosal, antibiotics, latex, gelatin, or formaldehyde	History of GBS within 6 weeks of previous influenza vaccination

Table 17 CONTINUED

Vaccine	Contraindications	Precautions
Influenza, live, attenuated (LAIV)	• People younger than 2 years or older than 49 years	• History of GBS within 6 weeks of previous influenza vaccination
	• Concomitant use of aspirin or aspirin-containing medication in children or adolescents through age 17 years	• Asthma in persons aged 5 years and older
	• Specific populations: pregnant women; immunosuppressed people; children ages 2 through 4 years who have asthma or had wheezing within the past 12 months; people who have taken influenza antiviral medications (amantadine, rimantadine, zanamivir, or oseltamivir) within the previous 48 hours; avoid using these antiviral agents for 14 days after vaccination	• Other chronic medical conditions (other chronic lung diseases; chronic cardiovascular diseases excluding isolated hypertension; diabetes; chronic renal or hepatitis disease; hematologic disease; neurologic disease; and metabolic disorders

(continued)

Table 17 CONTINUED

Vaccine	Contraindications	Precautions
Measles, mumps, rubella (MMR)—live	• Known severe immunodeficiency (e.g., from hematologic and solid tumors, receipt of chemotherapy, congenital immunodeficiency, or long-term immunosuppressive therapy, or patients with HIV infection who are severely immunocompromised • Pregnancy	• Recent (within 11 months) receipt of antibody-containing blood product (specific interval depends on product) • History of thrombocytopenia or thrombocytopenia purpura • Need for tuberculin skin testing (Measles vaccine may suppress tuberculin reactivity temporarily. MMR may be administered on the same day as tuberculin skin testing; however, if testing cannot be performed at the same time, the test should be postponed for at least 4 weeks after MMR vaccination.)
Pneumococcal conjugate (PCV13)	Severe allergic reaction (e.g., anaphylaxis) to any vaccine containing diphtheria toxoid	---
Rotavirus—live, attenuated oral RV5—RotaTeq RV1—Rotarix	• Severe combined immunodeficiency (SCID) • History of intussusception	• Immunodeficiency other than SCID • Chronic gastrointestinal disease## • Spina bifida or bladder extrophy##

Table 17 CONTINUED

Vaccine	Contraindications	Precautions
Varicella (VZV)—live	• Known severe immunodeficiency (e.g., from hematologic and solid tumors, receipt of chemotherapy, congenital immunodeficiency, or long-term immunosuppressive therapy, or patients with HIV infection who are severely immunocompromised) • Pregnancy	• Recent (within 11 months) receipt of antibody-containing blood product (specific interval depends on product)# • Receipt of specific antivirals (e.g., acyclovir, famiciclovir, or valacyclovir) 24 hours before vaccination; avoid use of these antiviral drugs for 14 days after vaccination
Zoster (HZV)—live	• Known severe cellular immunodeficiency (e.g., from hematologic and solid tumors, receipt of chemotherapy, congenital immunodeficiency, or long-term immunosuppressive therapy, or patients with HIV infection who are severely immunocompromised) • Pregnancy	• Receipt of specific antivirals (e.g., acyclovir, famiciclovir, or valacyclovir) 24 hours before vaccination; avoid use of these antiviral drugs for 14 days after vaccination

PART IV

TRAVEL VACCINES

YELLOW FEVER VACCINE

Did you know that:

- The earliest recorded record of yellow fever comes from a Mayan manuscript discovered in the Yucatan from 1648.
- Yellow fever was a major problem in the 18th century in colonial settlements in the Americas and West Africa. The disease was repeatedly introduced into seaports in the United States via sailing vessels infested with *Aedes aegypti* mosquitos that sustained transmission among the passengers and crew.
- In 1793 an outbreak of yellow fever in Philadelphia, which at the time was the federal capital of the United States, killed 10% of the population.
- The sweat of a person with yellow fever reportedly smells like a butcher's shop.

Yellow fever (YF) is transmitted in forested areas of sub-Saharan Africa and South America but may spread to urban areas and in dry locations where stored water provides breeding sites. Figure 8 shows the areas of the world where YF is endemic. YF illness ranges in severity from a self-limited, febrile illness to

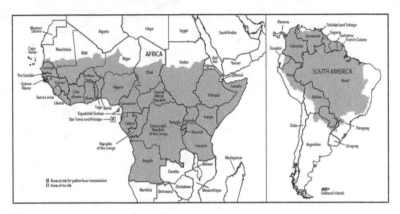

Figure 8   Areas requiring yellow fever vaccination

hemorrhagic fever that is fatal in 50% of cases. Up to 50% of infections are asymptomatic. After an incubation period of 3 to 6 days, fever, headache, and myalgias begin abruptly, accompanied by conjunctival injection, facial flushing, relative bradycardia, and leukopenia. In most cases these symptoms resolve with no further complications. In severe cases, after a short period of resolution, the symptoms return with high fever, headache, back pain, nausea, vomiting, abdominal pain, and somnolence. This is followed by severe weakness, icteric hepatitis, and prominent gastrointestinal bleeding, hematemesis, epistaxis, gum bleeding, and petechial and purpuric hemorrhages. Ultimately hypotension, shock, and metabolic acidosis develop accompanied by myocardial dysfunction, arrhythmias, azotemia, confusion, seizures, and coma. Death may occur within 7 to 10 days. A traveler's risk for acquiring yellow fever is determined by various factors, including immunization status, location of travel, season, duration of exposure, occupational and recreational activities while traveling, and local rate of virus transmission at the time of travel. From 1970 through 2013, a total of 10 cases of yellow fever were reported in unvaccinated travelers from the United States and Europe who traveled to West Africa (5 cases) or South America (5 cases). Eight (80%) of these 10 travelers died. The risk of acquiring yellow fever is difficult to predict because of variations in ecologic determinants of virus transmission. For a 2-week stay, the estimated risks for illness and death due to yellow fever for an unvaccinated traveler visiting an endemic area in:

- West Africa are 50 per 100,000 and 10 per 100,000, respectively
- South America are 5 per 100,000 and 1 per 100,000, respectively

Transmission

YF is transmitted by *Aedes aegypti* mosquitoes; the mosquitoes are infected after feeding on viremic humans and then spread the infection during subsequent feedings.

Incubation period

3 to 6 days after bite from infected mosquito

Treatment

No antiviral therapy is available. Treatment is supportive care.

Prevention

Preexposure prophylaxis
Yellow fever vaccine—live, attenuated 17D vaccine that is administered subcutaneously as single dose. Vaccine should be administered at least 10 days prior to travel. Compulsory vaccine is

required by certain countries for entry and can only be administered by certified travel clinics. Vaccine may be administered with other live vaccines. If not given at the same time, other live vaccines should be given 3 weeks later.

Duration of immunity

Probably lifelong after 1 dose, however, a booster dose is recommended every 10 years if a person resides or frequently travels to an endemic area.

Contraindications and precautions to yellow fever vaccine

Contraindications

1. Immunocompromised host
2. Anaphylactic reaction to eggs/egg products or prior dose of vaccine and any of its components
3. Age younger than 6 months, except during epidemics.

Precautions

1. Infants between 6 and 9 months of age and persons ≥ 60 years of age due to a very small increased risk of post-vaccination encephalitis (1 person in 125,000).
2. Pregnancy—not recommended unless travel to a high-risk endemic area cannot be avoided or postponed. In areas where YF is endemic, or during outbreaks, the benefits of YF vaccination are likely to far outweigh the risk of potential transmission of vaccine virus to the fetus or infant. Pregnant women and nursing mothers should be

counseled on the potential benefits and risks of vaccination so that they may make an informed decision about vaccination.

3. Breastfeeding—lactating women should be advised that the benefits of breastfeeding far outweigh alternatives. Vaccination is recommended, if indicated, for breastfeeding women traveling to endemic areas when such travel cannot be avoided or postponed or during epidemics.

Frequently asked questions

Does a patient need to avoid contact with immunocompromised family members after receiving the yellow fever vaccine?

No. There is no evidence that people who receive yellow fever vaccine shed the vaccine virus. Therefore, there is no need to avoid contact with persons who have weak immune systems.

How long should a woman wait to conceive after receiving a yellow fever vaccination?

Yellow fever vaccination has not been known to cause any birth defects when given to pregnant women and has been given to many pregnant women without any apparent adverse effects on the fetus. However, since yellow fever vaccine is a live virus vaccine, it poses a theoretical risk. While a two-week delay between yellow fever vaccination and conception is probably adequate, a 1-month delay has been advocated as a more conservative approach. If a woman is inadvertently or of necessity vaccinated during pregnancy, she is unlikely to have any problems from the vaccine and her baby is very likely to be born healthy.

Why is yellow fever vaccine not recommended to be given to adults 60 years and older even if they are traveling to an endemic area of the world?

People aged ≥60 years may be at increased risk for serious adverse events (serious disease or, very rarely, death) following vaccination, compared with younger persons. This is particularly true if they are receiving their first yellow fever vaccination. Travelers aged ≥60 years should discuss with their health-care provider the risks and benefits of the vaccine given their travel plans. In addition to considering the vaccine, travelers to endemic areas should protect themselves from yellow fever and other vector-borne diseases. Preventive measures include wearing clothes with long sleeves and long pants and using an effective insect repellent such as those with DEET, picaridin, IR3535, or oil of lemon eucalyptus.

TYPHOID FEVER VACCINE

Did you know that:

- Mary Mallon (a.k.a. "Typhoid Mary") immigrated from a small village in Northern Ireland in 1883 and served as a cook to wealthy families in New York City. She was responsible for at least 2 separate typhoid fever outbreaks resulting in infection of 51 persons and 3 deaths. Her poor hand hygiene caused her to spread disease so effectively.
- Typhoid Mary spent a total of 26 years in forced isolation to prevent the spread of the disease. She died in 1938 while still in isolation.
- Typhoid Mary was the first person in the United States identified as an asymptomatic carrier of the typhoid fever organism.

- Wolfgang Amadeus Mozart suffered from smallpox and a bout of typhoid fever during his lifetime.
- The sweat of a person with typhoid fever smells like freshly baked bread.

Typhoid fever is a global health problem with an estimated 26.9 million cases worldwide and 220,000 deaths each year. The disease is very common in developing countries, especially in the Indian subcontinent (India and Pakistan), Southeast Asia, South and Central America, and Africa. It is caused by several typhoidal *Salmonella* species, including *S. typhi*, *S. enterica* subtype enteritidis, and *S. paratyphi*. The onset of disease is gradual with symptoms ranging from mild to severe. The most common manifestations are high fever, headache, malaise, anorexia, lethargy, abdominal tenderness, hepatosplenomegaly, diarrhea or constipation, rose-colored spots on the trunk or abdomen, and changes in mental status. Persons with typhoid fever may excrete *Salmonella* organisms in their stools for months after having typhoid fever. This serves as a source of infection to their contacts. Complications may occur in up to 15% of patients. The most common complications include: GI bleeding, intestinal perforation, hepatitis, and encephalopathy. Five to 10% of patients will relapse even after receiving appropriate therapy.

Transmission

Acquisition of infection occurs by ingestion of fecally contaminated food or water (e.g., through handling by a person who is shedding *S. typhi* or if sewage contaminates the water used for drinking or washing food). Therefore, typhoid fever is more common in areas of the world where proper handwashing is less frequent and water is likely to be contaminated with sewage.

Incubation period

Incubation period is on average 8 to 14 days but ranges from 3 to 60 days or more.

Treatment

Response to antibiotic therapy is slow, and fever may persist for many days and even weeks after the patient's blood culture has cleared. Third-generation cephalosporins, azithromycin, and fluoroquinolones are first-line antibiotics.

Prevention

Preexposure prophylaxis
Vaccine dosage and delivery are summarized in Table 18.

Contraindications and precautions for typhoid fever vaccine

Contraindications
1. Persons with history of anaphylaxis after previous administration of the vaccine and in persons with suspected or proven hypersensitivity to any component of the vaccine.
2. For oral live, attenuated vaccine:
    i. Pregnancy
    ii. Individuals with an acute gastrointestinal condition or inflammatory bowel disease
    iii. Persons with known or suspected immunocompromising condition

Table 18 TYPHOID FEVER VACCINES

Vaccine name	Type of vaccine	How given	Number of doses necessary	Time between doses	Time immunization should be completed by (before possible exposure)	Minimum age for vaccination	Booster needed every…
Ty21a (Vivotif Berna, Swiss Serum and Vaccine Institute)	Live, attenuated, oral	PO—by mouth	4	2 days	1 week	6 years	5 years
ViCPS (Typhim Vi, Pasteur Merieux)	Inactivated	IM—Injection	1	N/A	2 weeks	2 years	2 years

Precautions
1. Persons with severe acute illness with or without fever
2. For oral live, attenuated vaccine:
    i. Persons who are taking antibiotics or certain antima-
    larials that may kill the organism in the vaccine.

Frequently asked questions

How long can an infected person carry the typhoid fever bacteria?
The duration of the carrier stage varies from days to years. Only about 3% of patients go on to become lifelong carriers and this tends to occur more often in adults than in children.

One of my relatives returned from a trip to Pakistan and has typhoid fever. Should my relative be kept away from other family members when they return home?
Only people with active diarrhea who are unable to control their bowels (e.g., infants, certain disabled individuals, persons with copious diarrhea) should be isolated. Most infected people may return to work or school when they have been appropriately treated with antibiotics, provided they carefully wash their hands after using the toilet. Children in daycare should obtain approval from the Department of Public Health before returning to their routine activities. Food handlers and those who provide patient care *may not* return to work until three consecutive negative stool specimens are obtained.

JAPANESE ENCEPHALITIS VACCINE

Did you know that:

- Mosquito larvae infected with the Japanese encephalitis virus are found in flooded rice fields, marshes, and small stable collections of water around cultivated fields. Pigs and certain species of wild birds actually amplify the virus in their bloodstreams when bitten, so areas where these animals are prevalent are areas of highest risk. Habitats supporting the transmission cycle of JE virus are principally in rural, pig farming, and rice paddy locations. Traveling and living "off the grid" in these locations places one at high risk for contracting this disease.
- Seizures with the disease occur in over 75% of pediatric patients but much less frequently in adults.

Japanese encephalitis (JE) virus is a Flavivirus that is an arthropod borne infection. It is transmitted in Asia over an area spanning one third of the world's circumference, from Pakistan at the westernmost edge to far eastern Russia. The disease is endemic and epidemic in Southeast Asia, China, and the Asian subcontinent, including Indonesian and the Philippines (see Figure 9 for endemic areas). Most infections with JE virus are asymptomatic. In countries where disease is endemic, infections acquired naturally at an early age results in immunity in over 80% of young adults. Symptomatic infections occur primarily in children between 2 and 10 years of age with higher incidence in males. Travelers of *all* ages without naturally acquired protective antibodies are at risk for

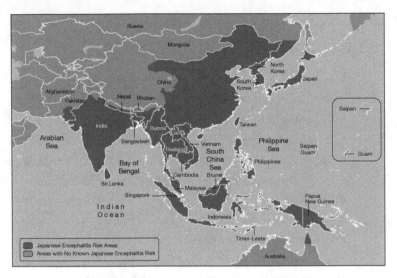

Figure 9 Map showing endemic areas for Japanese encephalitis

acquisition of the illness. Infection is symptomatic in less than 1% of cases of JE, but the illness usually presents as a severe encephalitis, leading frequently to coma and to a fatal outcome in 25% of cases.

The earliest symptoms are lethargy, fever, headache, abdominal pain, nausea, and vomiting. Lethargy increases over several days associated with agitated delirium, unsteadiness, and abnormal motor movements, advancing to progressive somnolence and coma. Multiple seizures and status epilepticus are associated with a poor outcome. Neurologic abnormalities persist in up to one-third of patients. A large proportion of recovered children (up to 75%), exhibit behavioral and psychological abnormalities. Illness acquired in the first and second trimesters of pregnancy may precipitate abortion.

Incubation

Incubation period is 5 to 15 days after being bitten by an infected mosquito.

Transmission

The virus is transmitted by the *Culex tritaeniorhynchus* and related ground-pool-breeding mosquitoes to pigs and aquatic birds, which are the principal viral amplifying hosts. Viremic adult pigs are asymptomatic, but infected pregnant sows abort or deliver stillbirths. Infected horses and humans are symptomatic. Rice paddies provide favorable breeding habitats for vector mosquitoes: therefore, the risk of infection is highest in rural areas with rice growing, pig farming, and horses, especially if the traveler is staying this area for more than 3 weeks.

Travelers at the highest risk are those who will be staying in rural rice-growing and pig-farming endemic areas for at least 3 weeks, engaging in extensive outdoor activities (e.g., camping, hiking, fishing, biking) in rural areas, and staying in accommodations that lack window screens, air conditioning, or bed nets.

Treatment

There is no specific therapy for JE encephalitis outside of supportive care.

Prevention

Preexposure prophylaxis
Japanese encephalitis vaccine: Ixaro is an inactivated vaccine that is a 2-dose series with doses given 28 days apart. Doses should be

completed at least 1 week prior to travel. It is licensed for use in persons ≥2 months of age. It is administered as:

A 0.5 ml IM dose to persons ≥3 years of age
A 0.25 ml IM dose to persons 2 months through 2 years of age.

Booster dose
Recommended for persons ≥17 years of age if continued exposure anticipated and greater than 1 year has elapsed since completion of the primary 2-dose series.

Contraindications and precautions for Japanese encephalitis vaccine

Contraindications
Severe allergic reaction (e.g., anaphylaxis) to a previous dose of vaccine or any vaccine component.

Precautions
1. Moderate or severe acute illness with or without fever.
2. Pregnancy—theoretical risk to the fetus, however, no deleterious effects have been demonstrated from JE vaccine administration during pregnancy, and the risk of adverse fetal effects from an inactivated vaccine is extremely low.

Duration of protection

Unknown

Frequently asked questions

Can a person get infected through close contact with an infected person?
No. JE virus has not been shown to be transmitted from person to person.

Can a person contract JE through eating pork that comes from an endemic area?
No. Once the pig is slaughtered the JE virus will not survive in the pork meat. JE virus can only survive in living cells. Any virus will be killed by cooking, roasting, or boiling the meat at a temperature of more than 60 degrees Celsius and the digestive enzymes and acid in our stomach will also kill the virus.

RABIES VACCINE

Did you know that:

- The earliest reported description of rabies is before 2300 BC in the Mesopotamian Laws of Eshnunna.
- Quote from Lewis Thomas in The Lives of a Cell, 1974: "I have seen agony in death only once, in a patient with rabies: he remained acutely aware of every stage in the process of his own disintegration over a twenty four-hour period, right up to his final moment."

Rabies is an acute illness with rapidly progressive central nervous system manifestations including anxiety, radicular pain, dysesthesia or pruritus, hydrophobia, and dysautonomia or paralysis. Illness almost invariably progresses to death. The disease has 3 sequential stages: (1) The prodromal stage, which lasts for 2 to 10 days and is characterized by fever, headache, malaise, fatigue, anorexia, anxiety, agitation, irritability, insomnia, depression, and pain, pruritus, or paresthesia at the site of the bite; (2) the acute neurologic state, which lasts 2 to 12 days, is characterized by hyperactivity, disorientation, hallucinations, bizarre behavior, aggressiveness, seizures, paralysis, aerophobia, hyperventilation, and cholinergic manifestations, including hypersalivation, lacrimation, mydriasis, and hyperpyrexia, with paralysis occuring in 20% of cases; (3) at the end of the neurologic stage, the patient may become comatose. Death from cardiorespiratory arrest usually occurs within 7 days, although with supportive care, coma may last for months. Each year, there are an estimated 70,000 human rabies cases worldwide, with only 1 to 2 cases occurring in the United States. Disease is almost always fatal.

Transmission

The virus is present in the saliva of a number of different animals and is transmitted by bites or by contamination of mucosa or skin lesions by saliva or other potentially infectious material. In the United States, bats, raccoons, skunks, foxes, wolves, coyotes, and bobcats, are the most important sources of infection for humans and domestic animals. Worldwide, most human cases of rabies result from dog or cat bites. Transmission also has occurred by transplantation of organs, corneas, and other tissues from patients dying of undiagnosed rabies.

Incubation period

The incubation period is 1 to 3 months but ranges from days to years.

Treatment

There is no specific treatment.

Prevention

Post-exposure

a. Post-exposure prophylaxis is recommended for all persons bitten by wild mammalian carnivores or bats or by domestic animals that are suspected to be rabid. It is also recommended for people who report an open wound, scratch, or mucous membrane that has been contaminated with saliva or other potentially infectious material from a rabid animal.

b. The injury inflicted by a bat bite or scratch may be small and not readily evident, or the circumstances of contact with a bat may preclude accurate recall (e.g., a bat in a room of a deeply sleeping or medicated person, or an unattended child, especially an infant or toddler who cannot reliably communicate about a potential bite). Therefore, postexposure prophylaxis may be indicated, for situations in which a bat physically is present in the same room if a bite or mucous membrane exposure cannot reliably be excluded, unless prompt testing of the bat has excluded rabies virus infection. **Prophylaxis should be initiated as soon as possible after bites by known or suspected rabid animals**.

c. The immediate objective of postexposure prophylaxis is to prevent virus from entering neural tissue. Prompt and thorough local treatment of all lesions is essential because virus may remain localized to the area of the bite for a variable time. All wounds should be flushed thoroughly and cleaned with soap and water. **After wound care is completed, concurrent use of passive and active prophylaxis is optimal.** The exception is in persons who previously have received complete vaccination regimens with a cell culture vaccine or people who have been vaccinated with other types of rabies vaccines and have previously had a documented rabies virus-neutralizing antibody titer; these people should receive only vaccine.

d. Prophylaxis should begin as soon as possible after exposure, **ideally within 24 hours.** However, a delay of several days or more may not compromise effectiveness, and **prophylaxis should be initiated if reasonably indicated, regardless of the interval between exposure and initiation of therapy.**

Passive prophylaxis—rabies immune globulin (RIG)—in the United States, only human RIG is available. The dosing is 20 IU/kg—wound site should be infiltrated with as much of the RIG as possible and any remaining volume should be administered intramuscularly. This should be used concomitantly with the first dose of vaccine to bridge the time between possible infection and antibody production induced by the vaccine.

Active prophylaxis—Human diploid cell vaccine (Imovax) and purified chicken embryo cell vaccine (RabAvert) are available for use in the United States.

a. For a previously unvaccinated immunocompetent person, a 1.0 ml dose of vaccine is given IM in the deltoid area (the anterolateral aspect of the thigh is also acceptable for children) on the first day of postexposure prophylaxis (Day 0), and repeated doses are given on days 3, 7, and 14 after the first dose for a total of 4 doses, with one dose of RIG given on day 0.

b. For a person with altered immunocompetence, postexposure prophylaxis should include a 5-dose vaccination regimen (i.e., 1 dose of vaccine on days 0, 3, 7, 14, and 28), with 1 dose of RIG on day 0.

Preexposure

a. Preexposure prophylaxis is recommended for people in high-risk groups, including veterinarians, animal handlers, certain laboratory workers, and people moving or traveling to areas where canine rabies is common. Others, such as spelunkers (cavers) or animal rehabilitators, who may have frequent exposures to bats and other wildlife, should also be considered for preexposure prophylaxis.

b. The preexposure prophylaxis vaccine schedule is a 3-dose series given as a 1.0 mL IM injection on days 0, 7, and 21 or 28.

Duration of protection

Serum antibodies usually persist for 2 years or longer after the primary series is administered IM.

Contraindications and precautions for rabies vaccine

Contraindications
In the situation of exposure to rabies, there are no contraindications to vaccination or use of HRIG.

Precautions

1. Severe allergic reaction (e.g., anaphylaxis) to a previous dose of vaccine or any vaccine component.

2. Immunosuppression—immunosuppressive agents should not be administered during postexposure prophylaxis unless absolutely essential. If possible, preexposure prophylaxis should be postponed until immunocompromising conditions are resolved. When an immunosuppressed person is given pre- or postexposure prophylaxis, antibody titers should be checked.

3. Patients with selective IgA deficiency may be at increased risk for anaphylactic reactions to HRIG because it may contain trace amounts of IgA.

Frequently asked questions

My granddaughter just received two hamsters for her birthday. Can these small rodents transmit rabies to humans?
Rabies in small rodents (e.g., squirrels, hamsters, guinea pigs, gerbils, chipmunks, rats, and mice) and lagomorphs such as rabbits, pikas, and hares is very rare and do not pose a rabies infection risk.

Is it possible to develop rabies from the rabies vaccine?
No, all rabies vaccines used in humans are inactivated and therefore it is not possible for the vaccine to cause disease.

CHOLERA VACCINE

Did you know that:

- Reports of cholera-like disease have been found as early as 1000 AD.

- Cholera has the distinction of being among the most rapidly fatal infectious diseases of humans with the ability to cause death within 6 to 12 hours of onset of clinical symptoms.
- Prior to the development of effective rehydration therapy with intravenous and oral fluids, cholera epidemics were associated with case-fatality rates that exceeded 60% and led to tens of thousands of deaths.
- The diarrhea of cholera is described as "rice-water stool." The stools are watery and often contain flecks of whitish material (mucus and some gastrointestinal lining cells) that are about the size of pieces of rice and smells "fishy."
- The volume of diarrhea can be enormous with as much as 250 cc per kg or about 10 to 18 liters of diarrhea fluid lost over a 24-hour period.

Cholera is an acute, rapidly dehydrating, watery, painless diarrheal disease caused by infection with toxogenic strains of the bacterium *Vibrio cholerae* serogroups O1 and O139. Serogroup O1 is the most common. The World Health Organization estimates that about 3 to 5 million people are infected worldwide each year, with approximately 100,000 deaths per year. Figure 10 shows the areas of the world where cholera outbreaks continue to be a problem. Cholera is now endemic in over 50 countries and can appear in explosive epidemics. Since the early 1800s, there have been 7 cholera pandemics. The current pandemic began in 1961 and is caused by *V. cholerae* O1 El Tor.

Cholera manifests as an acute, severe watery, painless diarrhea that can lead to death from dehydration within hours of onset. The spectrum of disease ranges from asymptomatic intestinal colonization (observed in individuals with preexisting immunity) to mild, moderate, and severe diarrhea. In severe diarrhea, the

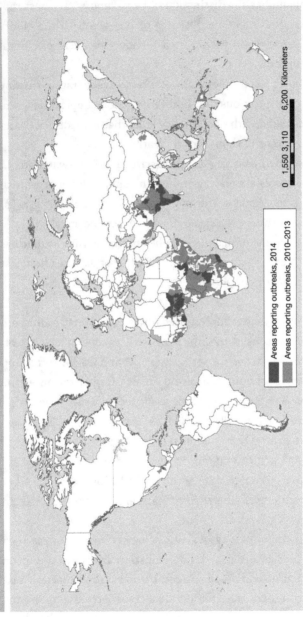

Cholera, areas reporting outbreaks, 2010–2014

Areas reporting outbreaks, 2014
Areas reporting outbreaks, 2010–2013

0   1,550 3,110   6,200 Kilometers

The boundaries and names shown and the designations used on this map do not imply the expression of any opinion whatsoever on the part of the World Health Organization concerning the legal status of any country, territory, city or area or of its authorities, or concerning the delimitation of its frontiers or boundaries. Dotted and dashed lines on maps represent approximate border lines for which there may not yet be full agreement.

Data Source: World Health Organization
Map Production: Health Statistics and Information Systems (HSI)
World Health Organization

World Health Organization

Figure 10 Cholera, areas reporting outbreaks 2010–2014

volume of watery stool can exceed 1L/hour. Vomiting is common, however, and patients are usually afebrile. As the dehydration worsens, patients may also experience muscle pain and spasm. In addition to potentially life-threatening dehydration and hypovolemia, common complications of cholera include hypokalemia, metabolic acidosis, and hypoglycemia.

Transmission

Transmission occurs through the consumption of contaminated water or food (especially raw or undercooked shellfish, raw or partially dried fish, or moist grains or vegetables stored at ambient temperature) and is often the result of a combined contamination. For example, contaminated water is often used to wash fresh food therefore contaminating the food. Spread of the infection is by the fecal-oral route and is associated with inadequate sanitation and unsafe water.

Incubation period

The incubation period is 1 to 3 days with a range of a few hours to 5 days.

Treatment

a. The cornerstone of management is appropriate rehydration therapy. Rehydration therapy should be based on WHO standards, with the goal of replacing the estimated fluid deficit within 3 to 4 hours of initial presentation. In patients with severe dehydration, isotonic intravenous fluids should be used, and lactated Ringer solution is the preferred commercially available option. For patients

Table 19 ANTIBIOTICS FOR TREATMENT OF SUSPECTED CHOLERA

Antibiotic	Pediatric Dose	Adult Dose
Azithromycin	20 mg/kg, single dose	1 gram, single dose
Ciprofloxacin*	15 mg/kg, twice daily X 3 days	500 mg, twice daily X 3 days
Doxycycline**	4–6 mg/kg, single dose	300 mg, single dose
Erythromycin	12.5 mg/kg, 4 times/day X 3 days	250 mg, 4 times/day X 3 days
Tetracycline	12.5 mg/kg, 4 times/day X 3 days	500 mg, 4 times/day X 3 days

*Ciprofloxacin is not recommended in children or pregnant women
** Doxycycline is not recommended in children younger than 8 years or in pregnant women

without severe dehydration, oral rehydration solution is the standard.

b. Prompt initiation of antimicrobial therapy decreases the duration and volume of diarrhea and decreases the shedding of viable bacteria. Antimicrobial therapy is recommended only for people who are moderately to severely ill. Table 19 shows the antibiotics for treatment of suspected cholera.

Prevention

a. A cholera vaccine (Vaxchora) was recently approved by the FDA for use in the United States. Preexposure prophylaxis is recommended for persons 18 to 64 years of age traveling to cholera-affected countries.

b. The vaccine is a live, attenuated vaccine that is taken as a single, oral liquid dose (~3 fl oz) at least 10 days prior to traveling to a cholera-affected area to protect against disease caused by *V. cholerae* serogroup O1.

c. Most common reported adverse reactions were tiredness, headache, abdominal pain, nausea/vomiting, lack of appetite, and diarrhea.

Duration of protection and efficacy

Unknown. Based on data from randomized, placebo controlled human challenge studies (challenged by oral ingestion of *V. cholerae*) the vaccine demonstrated an efficacy of 90.3% among persons challenged 10 days post-vaccination and 80% among those challenged 3 months post-vaccination.

Contraindications and precautions for cholera vaccine

Contraindications
Persons with a history of severe allergic reaction (e.g., anaphylaxis) to any ingredient of this cholera vaccine or to a previous dose of any cholera vaccine.

Precautions
1. The safety and effectiveness has not been established in immunocompromised persons or persons receiving immunosuppressive therapies. Vaccine strain may be shed in the stool of recipients for at least 7 days. There is a potential for transmission of the vaccine strain to non-vaccinated close contacts.
2. The safety and effectiveness has not been established in children and adolescents younger than 18 years or in adults over 65 years.

Frequently asked questions

Where do cholera outbreaks occur?

Cholera outbreaks occur in areas where there are natural disasters or in situations where there is a loss of sanitary human waste disposal and lack of clean water and foods for people to eat. In developing countries, hunger can lead people to eat contaminated food and/or drink contaminated water which increases the risk for cholera to infect malnourished populations.

Are there persons that are at higher risk to become infected with cholera than others?

Yes. People who are malnourished or immune compromised and children aged 2 to 4 years are more likely to become infected. Also people with blood type O are twice as likely to develop cholera and people with achlorhydria (reduced acid secretion in the stomach) or persons taking medications to reduce stomach acid (e.g., H2 blockers) are more likely to develop cholera because stomach acid kills the cholera organism.

How contagious is cholera?

It takes about 100 million *V. cholerae* bacteria to infect a healthy adult. Because this number is so high, significant contamination of food or water is required to transmit the disease. In outbreaks, cholera causing bacteria become highly contagious indirectly and directly by the fecal-oral route because of widespread fecal contamination of food, water, and items like bedding and clothing.

REFERENCES

http://www.cdc.gov/vaccines/schedules/index.html

http://www.immunizationinfo.org

http://www.vaccineinformation.org

www.publichealth.org

American Academy of Pediatrics Committee on Infectious Diseases. Poliovirus. Pediatrics 2011;128(4):805–808.

American Academy of Pediatrics. In Kimberlin DW, Brady MT, Jackson MA, Long SS (Eds.), *Red Book: 2015 Report of the Committee on Infectious Diseases*. Elk Grove Village, IL; American Academy of Pediatrics; 2015.

CDC. http://www.cdc.gov/vaccines/hcp/adults/for-practice/standards/recommend.html

CDC. http://www.cdc.gov/vaccines/hcp/conversations/about-vacc-conversations.html

CDC. http://www.cdc.gov/vaccines/hcp/patient-ed/conversations/downloads/not-vacc-risks-color-office.pdf

CDC. www.gov/vaccines/adultstandards

CDC. A Comprehensive Immunization Strategy to Eliminate Transmission of Hepatitis B Virus Infection in the United States: Recommendations of the Advisory Committee on Immunization Practices (ACIP): Part 1—Immunization of infants, children, and adolescents. MMWR Morb Mortal Wkly Rep 2005;54(RR16):14.

CDC. A Comprehensive Immunization Strategy to Eliminate Transmission of Hepatitis B Virus Infection in the United States: Recommendations of the Advisory Committee on Immunization Practices (ACIP): Part 2—Immunization of adults. MMWR Morb Mortal Wkly Rep 2006;55(RR-16):13.

CDC. Epidemiology and Prevention of Vaccine Preventable Diseases—The Pink Book: Course Textbook. 13th Edition, 2015.

CDC and US Department of Health and Human Services. Guidelines for Vaccinating Pregnant Women. October 2012.

CDC. Advisory Committee on Immunization Practices Recommended Immunization Schedule for Children and Adolescents Aged 18 Years or Younger—United States, 2017. MMWR Morb Mortal Wkly Rep 2017;66(5):134–135.

CDC. Advisory Committee on Immunization Practices Recommended Immunization Schedule for Adults Aged 19 Years and Older—United States, 2017. MMWR Morb Mortal Wkly Rep 2017;66(5):136–138.

CDC. General Recommendations on Immunization: Recommendations of the Advisory Committee on Immunization Practices (ACIP). MMWR Morb Mortal Wkly Rep 2011;60(2):26–27.

CDC. Human Papillomavirus Vaccination: Recommendations of the Advisory Committee on Immunization Practices (ACIP). MMWR Morb Mortal Wkly Rep 2014;63(RR05):1–30.

CDC. Immunization of Health-Care Personnel: Recommendations of the Advisory Committee on Immunization Practices. MMWR Recommendations and Reports 2011;60(7):1–45.

CDC. Licensure of a Meningococcal Conjugate Vaccine for Children Aged 2 through 10 Years and Updated Booster Dose Guidance for Adolescents and Other Persons at Increased Risk for Meningococcal Disease—ACIP, 2011. MMWR Morb Mortal Wkly Rep 2011;60(30):1018–1019.

CDC. Preventing Tetanus, Diphtheria, and Pertussis Among Adolescents: Use of Tetanus Toxoid, Reduced Diphtheria Toxoid and Acellular Pertussis Vaccines: Recommendations of the Advisory Committee on Immunization Practices. MMWR Recommendations and Reports 2006;55(RR03):1–34.

CDC. Preventing Tetanus, Diphtheria, and Pertussis Among Adults: Use of Tetanus Toxoid, Reduced Diphtheria Toxoid and Acellular Pertussis Vaccines: Recommendations of the Advisory Committee on Immunization Practices, supported by the Healthcare Infection Control Practices Advisory Committee, for Use of Tdap Among Health-Care Personnel. MMWR Recommendations and Reports 2006;55(RR17):1–33.

CDC. Prevention of Hepatitis A Through Active or Passive Immunization: Recommendations of the Advisory Committee on Immunization Practices (ACIP). MMWR Morb Mortal Wkly Rep 2006;55(RR-7):15.

CDC. Prevention of varicella: recommendations of the Advisory Committee on Immunization Practices (ACIP). MMWR Morb Mortal Wkly Rep 2007;56(RR-4):28, 31.

CDC. Prevention of herpes zoster: recommendations of the Advisory Committee on Immunization Practices (ACIP). MMWR Morb Mortal Wkly Rep 2008;57(RR-5):21.

CDC. Prevention of Pneumococcal Disease Among Infants and Children— Use of 13-valent Pneumococcal Conjugate Vaccine and 23-valent Pneumococcal Polysaccharide Vaccine. MMWR Morb Mortal Wkly Rep 2010;59(RR-11):1–18.

CDC. Prevention of Measles, Rubella, Congenital Rubella Syndrome, and Mumps, 2013: Summary Recommendations of the Advisory Committee on Immunization Practices (ACIP). MMWR Morb Mortal Wkly Rep 2013;62(RR04):1–34.

CDC. Prevention and Control of Seasonal Influenza with Vaccines. Recommendations of the Advisory Committee on Immunization Practices—United States, 2016–17 Influenza Season. MMWR Morb Mortal Wkly Rep 2016;65(05):1–54.

CDC. Progress toward elimination of *Haemophilus influenzae* type b invasive disease among infants and children: United States, 1998–2000. MMWR Morb Mortal Wkly Rep 2002;51:234–237.

CDC. Progress Toward Polio Eradication—Worldwide, 2015–2016. MMWR Morb Mortal Wkly Rep 2016;65(18):470–473.

CDC. Recommendations for Use of Meningococcal Conjugate Vaccines in HIV Infected Persons—Advisory Committee on Immunization Practices, 2016. MMWR Morb Mortal Wkly Rep 2016;65(43):1189–1194.

CDC. Updated Recommendation from the Advisory Committee on Immunization Practices for Revaccination of Persons at Prolonged Increased Risk for Meningococcal Disease. MMWR Morb Mortal Wkly Rep 2009;58(37):1042–1043.

CDC. Updated Recommendations for Prevention of Invasive Pneumococcal Disease Among Adults Using the 23-valent Pneumococcal Polysaccharide Vaccine (PPSV23). MMWR Morb Mortal Wkly Rep 2010;59(34):1102–1106.

CDC. Updated Recommendations for Use of Tetanus Toxoid, Reduced Diphtheria Toxoid and Acellular Pertussis (Tdap) Vaccine from the Advisory Committee on Immunization Practices, 2010. MMWR Morb Mortal Wkly Rep 2011;60(1):13–15.

CDC. Updated Recommendations for Use of Tetanus Toxoid, Reduced Diphtheria Toxoid, and Acellular Pertussis (Tdap) Vaccine in Pregnant Women and Persons who have or Anticipate Having Close Contact with an Infant Aged <12 months—Advisory Committee on Immunization Practices (ACIP), 2011. MMWR Morb Mortal Wkly Rep 2011;60(41):1424–1426.

CDC. Updated Recommendations for Use of Tetanus Toxoid, Reduced Diphtheria Toxoid, and Acellular Pertussis (Tdap) Vaccine in Adults Aged 65 years and older—Advisory Committee on Immunization Practices (ACIP), 2012. MMWR Morb Mortal Wkly Rep 2012;61(25):468–470.

CDC. Updated Recommendations for Use of Tetanus Toxoid, Reduced Diphtheria Toxoid, and Acellular Pertussis Vaccine (Tdap) in Pregnant Women—Advisory Committee on Immunization Practices (ACIP), 2012. MMWR Morb Mortal Wkly Rep 2013;62(07):131–135.

CDC. Use of 13-Valent Pneumococcal Conjugate Vaccine and 23-Valent Pneumococcal Polysaccharide Vaccine for Adults with Immunocompromising Conditions: Recommendations of the ACIP. MMWR Morb Mortal Wkly Rep 2012;61(40):816–819.

CDC. Use of 13-Valent Pneumococcal Conjugate Vaccine and 23-Valent Pneumococcal Polysaccharide Vaccine Among Adults Aged ≥65 Years: Recommendations of the Advisory Committee on Immunization Practices (ACIP). MMWR Morb Mortal Wkly Rep 2014;63(37):822–825.

CDC. Use of a 2-Dose Schedule for Human Papillomavirus Vaccination—Updated Recommendations of the Advisory Committee on Immunization Practices. MMWR Morb Mortal Wkly Rep 2016;65(49):1405–1408.

CDC. Use of Serogroup B Meningococcal Vaccines in Adolescents and Young Adults: Recommendations of the Advisory Committee on Immunization Practices, 2015. MMWR Morb Mortal Wkly Rep 2015;64(4):1171–1176.

CDC. Use of Serogroup B Meningococcal Vaccines in Persons Ages ≥10 Years at Increased Risk for Serogroup B Meningococcal Disease: Recommendations of the Advisory Committee on Immunization Practices, 2015. MMWR Morb Mortal Wkly Rep 2015;64(22):608–612.

Dennehy PH. Effects of vaccine on rotavirus disease in the pediatric population. Curr Opin Pediatr 2012;24:76–84.

DeStefano F, Price CS, Weintraub ES. Increasing exposure to antibody-stimulating proteins and polysaccharides in vaccines is not associated with risk of autism. J Pediatr 2013;163:561–567.

Dube E, Laberge C, Guay M, et al. Vaccine hesitancy: an overview. Human Vac Immunother 2013;9(8):1763–1773.

Institute of Medicine. Adverse effects of Vaccines: Evidence and Causality. August 2011. Washington, DC: National Academics Press. At: www.iom.edu/vaccineadverseeffects

Institute of Medicine. Immunization Safety Review: Vaccines and Autism. May 2004. Washington, DC: National Academics Press. At: www.iom.nationalacademies.org

Offit PA, Jew RK. Addressing parents' concerns: Do vaccines contain harmful preservatives, adjuvants, additives, or residuals? Pediatrics 2003;112(6):1394–1401.

Offit PA, Quarles J, Gerber MA, et al. Addressing parents' concerns: Do multiple vaccines overwhelm or weaken the infant's immune system? Pediatrics 2002;109(1):124–129.

Rubin LG, et al. 2013 IDSA Clinical Practice Guidelines for Vaccination of the Immunocompromised Host. Clin Infect Dis 2014;58(3):e44–100.

Witteman HO. Addressing vaccine hesitancy with values. Pediatrics 2015;136(2).

INDEX

Note: Page numbers followed by f and t indicate figures and tables, respectively.